Incredible Raves for Fism,

"FISMAN'S FRAUD is both a disturbing and an exhilarating read. The book exposes what is effectively a crime scene with various agents complicit in producing fraudulent science that was used by media and the Prime Minister to fuel hatred and societal division.

Watteel reveals in precise detail how every system of oversight and accountability, from the University of Toronto to the Ontario Provincial Police failed in their duty to act with integrity. The exhilarating aspect is that the book shines a bright light on those responsible. Watteel names names and calls them out for what they are — morally bankrupt. Fisman's Fraud gives hope that by exposing the fraud justice may prevail and civility restored to this Nation."

— Ted Kuntz, President Vaccine Choice Canada

"FISMAN'S FRAUD is a must read that slices through the layers of lost integrity, accountability and responsibility to reveal the greatest deception of our time.

Easy to read but hard to swallow, the facts speak volumes in implicating those in power who intentionally failed to keep the ship off the rocks. Although the content is specific to Ontario, the implications were deadly, far-reaching and the situation warrants further investigation. Those responsible are currently still at the helm and the ship is in dangerous waters."

— Vincent A Gircys, Veteran Police Constable, Ontario Provincial Police - Forensic Collision Reconstructionist

FISMAN'S FRAUD

The Rise of
CANADIAN HATE SCIENCE

R.N. Watteel, PhD Statistics

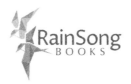

An Imprint of Whisperwood Publishing | Canada

This is a work of nonfiction. No names have been changed, no characters invented, no events fabricated. I am not a lawyer; views do not represent legal opinion. I have made every effort to ensure that the information in this book was correct at press time. Views are my own based on evidence as referenced in the book. Readers are encouraged to assess the evidence presented in order to draw their own conclusions.

FISMAN'S FRAUD

REPLACING REAL-WORLD OBSERVATIONS WITH A FICTIONAL SIMULATION IN AN ATTEMPT TO SCAPEGOAT AN UNPROTECTED MINORITY FOR PRODUCT FAILURE

PREFACE

Journey to Hell… and back? We'll see.

Before April 25th, 2022 I had little to no knowledge of David Fisman. I say "little to no knowledge" instead of "no knowledge" because, in all likelihood, his name had come up on the radio or in news articles that I'd stumbled upon without taking much notice. With so much profound upheaval over the course of the pandemic, bigger problems were top of mind. Well, all that changed one afternoon in spring after encountering numerous headlines warning of the risk of mixing with the "unvaccinated."

Instinctively and scientifically, I knew the headlines to be false, and so ignored them at first. I assumed the media was just sensationalizing yet another garbage study, one of many that had been published throughout the pandemic. But the headlines kept popping up everywhere, and the timing seemed suspicious given the politics at play. So, I pulled up the actual study to see first-hand how the researchers possibly could have arrived at such a backwards conclusion.

Utter disgust. That is the feeling that best sums up the experience. Disgust as a mathematician and statistician. Disgust as a mother. Disgust as a Canadian. Disgust as an honest and decent human being.

I couldn't believe what I was reading, initially flooded with so many thoughts and emotions. The nonsense of it all was dizzying. I had to walk away from the so-called "study" several times, midstream, just to clear my head. Appalling on so many levels, I haven't been able to let it go. Straightaway, I recognized the societal discord it was meant to sow and the hateful policies it was attempting to legitimize. I had become all too familiar with them. There was no way I could hold my tongue on this one. How could anyone?

Canadian hate science is not to be taken lightly.

To be fair, my journey to this point didn't start with the Fisman study — it started back in March 2020 when the Ontario government first announced a two-week shutdown to "flatten the curve." I recall entering the roundabout just ahead of my Starbucks exit. I nearly did a 360 back home, but I needed my caffeine, so I got my venti extra-hot latte to go. I rushed home, fired up my laptop and got to work gathering all the world-wide pandemic data I could get my hands on. I was determined to figure out what the hell was going on.

Foremost on my mind was to assess the risk the pandemic posed to family members so that we could take whatever precautionary measures might be necessary to ensure good health. I have four siblings, two of whom were in the medical profession — both working in hospital settings at the time. One sibling was a front-line respiratory therapist, another a cardiology technologist. I have ailing parents; my father suffers from several comorbid conditions including diabetes and congestive heart failure. My mother is a retired nurse. I have three children, one in high school and two in university. My husband works as a physicist for the federal government. Personally, I have no institutional affiliations. My career path as a principal statistician had taken an unexpected turn in my mid-thirties when a substance-impaired driver rammed into me, crushing my legs while loading groceries into the trunk of my car. I ultimately left my position to focus on rehabilitation, health and caring for my young family.

As for my background, I hold a PhD in statistics with a strong grounding in the sciences. I attained a Bachelor of Science degree from McMaster University. Studying in the Natural Sciences Program allowed me to take a wide spectrum of science courses before specializing in applied mathematics and theoretical physics. I went on to attain a Master of Science degree in the field of statistics before capping off my formal education at the University of Western Ontario.

I enjoyed working as a statistical sleuth throughout grad school and served as an independent consultant to medical practitioners, social scientists and afterwards to various levels of government. I also taught both undergraduate and graduate level statistics courses and developed an advanced-level course in data analysis. After moving to Ottawa, I served as senior, then principal, statistician for an economics consulting firm that specialized in risk-benefit and options analysis as well as program evaluation. Much of the work undertaken was for government departments at the municipal, provincial and federal levels, making me well-versed in their risk-management practices.

Compared to the assessments I had done in the past, the general risk analysis for COVID-19 was straightforward and the results markedly clear: the very elderly and those with comorbid conditions were at highest risk; healthy, working-aged individuals were at fairly low, manageable risk; while children and young adults had almost no risk of serious COVID-19 complications — less than the seasonal flu. Moreover, the risk between the oldest age group and the youngest changed by a factor of about a thousand. Based on this early assessment, my focus turned to my aging parents and my two siblings who worked in the health care sector. I kept track of the changing dynamics, government responses, emerging scientific findings as well as vaccine progress. When the clinical trial reports and assessments became available, I was quick to study them.

Things didn't add up right from the beginning. At every stage in the pandemic the government appeared to act nearly *opposite* to what the data indicated should be done, at least from a risk mitigation perspective. And when the vaccines rolled out, my concerns multiplied.

During the spring of 2021, I became increasingly concerned about the use of the novel vaccines on children and healthy young adults given the absence of long-term safety data or any clear benefits to them. In addition, concerns of myocarditis in youths had also been raised in the medical community. That summer, there was talk of mandatory vaccination for in-person university courses, health care workers and federal employees. From a risk-benefit perspective, I understood this to be a very dangerous precedent. So, when the 2021 federal election was called, in a protective impulse I threw my hat into the ring to oppose the mandates. Desperate times call for desperate measures, so the saying goes. I had no shot at winning, but I gave it my all, nonetheless, just to get the message out.

Sadly, the mandates came to pass. Hard months followed. The unvaccinated were barred from international travel, yet the Omicron variant made its way to Canada all the same. Unvaccinated Canadians weren't permitted to travel within their own country by plane or train, but cases surged across the provinces anyway. Workplaces that had purged their premises of unvaccinated workers saw an unprecedented rise in COVID-19 cases amongst their vaccinated workforce. COVID-19 cases rose to record heights, dwarfing all pre-vaccination peaks. Canadian COVID-19 hospitalizations under the milder cold-like variant more than doubled previous records. It became impossible to hide the complete failure of the vaccines to curtail community transmission, and equally difficult to interpret the segregation of the unvaccinated as anything but unfounded discrimination. Provinces soon abandoned their vaccine passports and by spring of 2022 it seemed the federal restrictions were ready to topple... That is, until Fisman's "study" miraculously appeared and gave the feds one last gasp for air.

Upon reading the Fisman (main author), Tuite and Amoako study in April 2022, I was astounded by the apparent ideologically driven bias, the blatantly fraudulent statements, and the call to action for punitive measures based on the faux analysis. I had never read such a problematic study — and I'm not alone in saying as much. Scientists around the globe were flabbergasted.

That such a study was published in a peer-reviewed science journal was both shocking and deeply worrisome. It seemed a new low in research had been attained. With so many media outlets running with the story and promoting societal division based on the false findings, it became abundantly clear that this fraudulent activity needed to be addressed. The study's potential to influence public policy and set an unacceptable precedent in the production, distribution and ultimate consumption of degenerate science had to be curtailed. So,

I reached out to the Canadian Medical Association Journal.
I wrote them ONCE. I wrote them TWICE. I wrote them THREE TIMES!

I reached out to the University of Toronto.
ONCE. TWICE. THREE TIMES!

I reached out to The Canadian Institutes of Health Research.
AM I INVISIBLE?

Deny. Deflect. Dismiss.

So, I wrote to the Ontario Provincial Police.
I requested an investigation and sent them a 150-page evidential report.

I wrote to the Premier's office.
I asked that they support an OPP investigation.

Lip service.

I can only assume they were all waiting for me to write a book.

Well, here it is.

CONTENTS

Chapter 1

Introduction

"It is pretty obvious that the debasement of the human mind caused by a constant flow of fraudulent advertising is no trivial thing. There is more than one way to conquer a country."
— *Raymond Chandler, American author (1888–1959)*

In December 2020, Canada ushered in its first-ever genetic vaccines to become widely available in response to the COVID-19 pandemic. Approval of these rushed-to-market injections was based on preliminary clinical trial results and an incomplete safety profile, with no mid- or long-term safety record. In the months that followed, tensions between the "vaccinated" and "unvaccinated" grew, fuelled by sensationalized media headlines and one-sided articles. By September 2021, "vaccine passports" had become a requirement to gain entry into restaurants, theatres, gyms, many university campuses and other public venues. Vaccination soon was mandatory for certain jobs in addition to travel by plane or train. Then, almost poetically, the Omicron wave hit and the shaky science behind the government-sanctioned vaccine passports and restrictions began to crumble. COVID-19 cases surged amongst the population, irrespective of vaccination status. "Follow the science" became code for "follow the groupthink."

On April 25th, 2022 a research study appeared in a respected Canadian medical journal claiming justification and strong support for federal and provincial restrictions based on vaccination status. It was David Fisman and his University of Toronto colleagues to the federal government's rescue.

> *"Vaccinated individuals have a right not to have their efforts to protect themselves undermined," Fisman said, stressing that the (study) findings are "very supportive" of vaccine mandates for flights and trains.*

> — *Forbes, April 25, 2022*[1]

The divisive study took Canada by storm. Its main author, David Fisman — an outspoken and partisan supporter of harsh public policy with numerous ties to the pharmaceutical industry — claimed that people who decline COVID-19 vaccination put the vaccinated at disproportionate risk.

Within hours of the study's official publication, articles in dozens of top newspapers and magazines flooded the nation, warning of the dire risks of merely "hanging out" with unvaccinated people. The vaccine was touted as powerful at stifling COVID-19, yet, it was incapable of protecting the population so long as the unvaccinated were present. Somehow, the absurd notion spread like wildfire.

Those who refused to accept the genetic injections were vilified as selfish souls. Numerous podcasts, interviews and articles citing Fisman's paper compared the unvaccinated to carriers of syphilis and reckless drivers.

Can't get an operation? Blame the unvaccinated! The "science" says so.

But did it?

This book examines the basis for the claims made by David Fisman and his two colleagues, Afia Amoako and Ashleigh R. Tuite. Evidence shows the researchers concocted a model simulation that FLIPPED reality, then proceeded to inform policy based on this inverted, false reality. More specifically, the study leveraged a false premise to support public policy aimed at enhancing vaccine uptake and limiting access to public spaces for unvaccinated people.

In essence, the researchers overwrote the Omicron surge with a fake simulation showing disproportionately greater infection rates amongst the unvaccinated — a trend opposite reality — in an attempt to scapegoat the unvaccinated for: 1) SARS-CoV-2 transmission, 2) vaccine failure, and 3) poor public health care decisions. But the research trio went even further.

The three career mathematical modellers proceeded to pass off the fabricated results as fact despite no real data being used, no hypothesis being tested and no model validation of any kind. Under the guise of "science" the researchers claimed the results supported the governments' harsh vaccine restrictions. When called out by troves of researchers from around the world for the flawed modelling and deceptive findings, the researchers refused to correct the record. Instead, the main author doubled-down on his divisive rhetoric and support of punitive measures against the unvaccinated.

Fabrication and falsification of data and results are two of the most severe violations of research integrity. They constitute intentional research fraud, violate fundamental research standards and defy basic societal values. The researchers used their position of trust in the community to push a harmful narrative, one that incites division and hate against an unprotected, vulnerable group that has been the target of extreme political castigation.

About This Book

Fisman's fraud extends well beyond the norms of science, attacking the very fabric of society. On their own, the three researchers would have had little influence. But they, along with others beholden to the same agenda, have been afforded a lofty platform to promote their faux science and to sow discord.

The main objectives of this book are to: (1) present evidence of the scientific misconduct, (2) convey the serious ramifications of such malfeasance, (3) expose the establishment's willingness to back knowingly fraudulent research that promotes disinformation and division, and (4) demonstrate the need for action.

The evidence presented herein shows that the conduct in question is not a matter of unwitting incompetence or a mere difference in scientific opinion. The acts were deliberate, ongoing and appear to have been part of a greater web of complicity. Moreover, there is reason to believe that this is just the beginning.

Given the stakes, it is important to seek accountability and to deter others from weaponizing science to persecute and oppress others.

CHAPTER 2

Web of Complicity

"Oh what a tangled web we weave when first we practice to deceive."
— *Sir Walter Scott, Scottish author (1771–1832)*

What is a Fact?

A fact (Collins English Dictionary): (1) an event or thing known to have happened or existed, (2) a truth verifiable from experience or observation.[2]

The Merriam-Webster definition is similar: A fact refers to an actual occurrence or a piece of information that has objective reality.[3] But then, one may ask: What is real? —*Real, as in not imagined, supposed, invented or theoretical.*

The basic concept of what constitutes a fact is central to this book. There should be no need to define such a basic construct here, but it appears many individuals rather suddenly have lost the ability to distinguish between what constitutes a fact and what does not. Even more worrisome, it seems that many in society specifically tasked with distinguishing between fact and opinion have not been spared this terrible disorder.

So to be clear, a fact is a thing that is known or proven to be true. It is not speculation, an opinion, or a matter of interpretation.

Have researchers also been stricken with this puzzling affliction? Perhaps some. Others may very well be the cause. Consider the case of Dr. David Fisman, Dr. Ashleigh Tuite, and Afia Amoako who presented their fictional results as scientific fact.

The research trio concocted a faux scientific model to fabricate data indicating that those people who opt out of COVID-19 vaccination (the "unvaccinated") constitute a disproportionate risk to the vaccinated population, a trend contrary to reality. These fabricated results were presented as facts and published by the Canadian Medical Association Journal (CMAJ). The authors then used this false claim to advocate for public health policies restricting unvaccinated people's access to public spaces along with harsh public actions to coerce vaccine uptake.

The University of Toronto trio, David Fisman, Afia Amoako and Ashleigh R. Tuite, conducted fraudulent research, funded by the Canadian Institutes of Health Research, then proceeded to present the fabricated results as scientific fact in order to inform government policy seeking to defraud millions of Canadians of basic rights and freedoms.

The findings were slopped up by dozens of media outlets warning of the risks of mingling with those reckless, syphilis carrying motorists, "the unvaccinated." The news even entered into Canadian parliamentary proceedings just a few days later. A timely development — the Trudeau government was in desperate need of "scientific" justification for extending their federal vaccine mandates and travel restrictions, irrespective of the vaccines' utter failure to curb Omicron.

Unfortunately, my many attempts to have the massive errors contained within the study corrected by the researchers were unsuccessful. However, in the process I have uncovered evidence pointing to a deeper network of support for the misconduct and academic malfeasance.

The Players & the Politics

It is clear the researchers did not act alone. Three organizations were directly connected to the study: (1) the Canadian Medical Association Journal (CMAJ) — the journal that published the study; (2) the University of Toronto (U of T) — the institution where the research was carried out; and (3) the Canadian Institutes of Health Research (CIHR) — the federal institution that funded the study. All three institutions were sent letters requesting an investigation into allegations of research misconduct along with supporting evidence and a detailed account of the study's many other critical flaws. Figure 1 illustrates the progression of my complaints against the Fisman et al. study and correspondences with the three institutions.

Canadian Medical Association Journal

Unexpectedly, my efforts to have the Fisman paper retracted and the record corrected revealed a web of complicity and self-serving interests. Incriminating changes made to the Fisman paper as it propagated through the CMAJ peer review process indicate that the journal was actively involved in the evolution of the deceptive and defamatory content.

Perhaps the most striking revisions involved efforts to present the illusion that the simulated trends were based on **real** people as opposed to predetermined results concocted by the researchers. With the elimination of modelling jargon together with repeated insertions of the word "people" — used only once in the preprint but appearing 76 times in the final publication — it's little wonder laypersons mistook the fake study for one grounded in reality.

The inclusion of unwarranted and derisive comparisons in the CMAJ publication was jarring for what should have been an objective scientific paper. Fisman, the lead author, subsequently engaged in numerous interviews, podcasts, and social media exchanges where he continued to exploit the fraudulent study and defame individuals. The defamatory statements included: casting the unvaccinated as casual spreaders of disease who constitute an unacceptable risk to other people; comparing the decision to not take the COVID-19 vaccines to reckless behaviour such as driving under the influence of alcohol and other intoxicants, or driving at 200 km/hr for fun; and, insinuating that the unvaccinated were largely

Figure 1: Flowchart of Complaint Progression Against Fisman, Tuite and Amoako

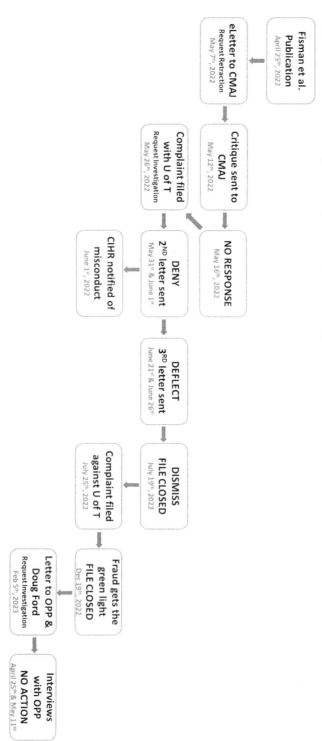

responsible for overburdening hospitals and causing the cancellation of elective surgeries for cancer and cardiac disease patients.

The defamatory statements were a clear effort to tarnish the character and reputation of the unvaccinated, to influence policy makers, and to seek public buy-in for punitive measures against the unvaccinated. I was shocked to discover that, far from screening out such statements, a number of them actually had been added *during* the peer review process.

There's little doubt that the modifications made to the preprint helped spur the media's sensationalized headlines. It is rare for academic papers to get such mainstream publicity. The publication's online engagement represented CMAJ's second most highly engaged article, as tracked by Altmetric Digital Science, since tracking began in 2011. It scored in the top 0.01% of all online research outputs across all sources.

Box 1: Online Engagement

As of April 6 2023:

> The study has been cited in at least 113 news stories from 90 outlets.

> The article scored higher than 99.99% of all research outputs across all sources.

> The article scored second place for online engagement of all CMAJ articles since 2011.

Additionally, the Fisman et al. publication received the most online engagement of all CMAJ articles within six weeks on either side of the publication date (as tracked by Altmetric Digital Science).[4]

A detailed examination of key revisions made from preprint to publication is provided later in the book (Chapter 9).

The material presented hereafter seeks to correct the record by demonstrating the falsity and harmful nature of the claims made by the research trio against those who chose not to take the novel genetic vaccines. Given the influence this research has had on public opinion, the main researcher's influence in shaping public policy, and the harm of allowing the rhetoric to continue unchallenged, it is my belief that it is in the public's best interest to expose the fraud.

University of Toronto: A Central Hub

As noted, the CMAJ study was co-authored by three University of Toronto researchers:

- **David Fisman** (lead author): A tenured professor in the Division of Epidemiology at University of Toronto's Dalla Lana School of Public Health.[5] One of his key areas of teaching and research is mathematical modelling of diseases to determine the rate at which people become infected with diseases. Fisman is also a medical doctor registered with the College of Physicians and Surgeons of Ontario (CPSO) for Internal Medicine;[6]

- **Ashleigh R. Tuite** (co-author): An assistant professor in the Division of Epidemiology at University of Toronto's Dalla Lana School of Public Health.[7] Ashleigh Tuite is an infectious disease epidemiologist and mathematical modeller; she holds a PhD in epidemiology and mathematical modelling as well as a Masters of Public Health. Ashleigh Tuite was employed by the Public Health Agency of Canada when the research was conducted; and

- **Afia Amoako** (co-author): A PhD student in epidemiology at the University of Toronto specializing in mathematical modelling techniques.

The University of Toronto has a solid domestic and international reputation. Not only is U of T a top-ranking Canadian university, it was ranked one of the world's top 20 schools according to the Times Higher Education World University Rankings, and a top-25 school in the QS World University Rankings and the Center for World University Rankings (CWUR, 2023). It ranked #21 overall (#15 in medicine) as the most influential university in the world according to AcademicInfluence.com (2022).

The university's first-rate reputation lends credibility to research published by its professors and affiliates. There is an expectation that complaints of research misconduct will be taken seriously. Sadly they are not, at least, not all of them.

I submitted a formal complaint to U of T calling for an investigation into allegations of research fraud. The allegations included fabrication and falsification of data and results; specific text-book incidents of the scientific fraud were highlighted. I followed U of T's process for dealing with such allegations. Their framework promises a thorough process to address and resolve all questions raised by the complaint.

The university had no interest whatsoever in investigating the misconduct. After a few back-and-forth letters prompting them to reconsider, U of T closed the file without addressing a single concern.

Why would a reputable organization stand behind such easily disproven research?

In April 2022, just weeks before Fisman's paper was released, the University of Toronto announced a partnership with Moderna Inc. to advance research in RNA science and technology.[8] The university supported COVID-19 vaccine mandates and restrictions throughout the pandemic and had, like many universities across the country, been granted large financial incentives from the Government of Canada to address "vaccine hesitancy" and other related matters.[9]

U of T required students and staff to show proof they'd been vaccinated to attend campus during the 2021/22 academic year. In the fall of 2022, months after the provincial vaccine passports were abandoned, the university reinstated and extended their vaccine requirements for those living in student residences, mandating at least three doses of a COVID-19 vaccine. They encouraged other universities to follow suit with similar policies.

As shown in the next chapter, the University of Toronto took on a central role during the pandemic, hosting the Ontario COVID-19 Science Advisory Table that advised the Ontario government's pandemic response. The table itself was predominantly comprised of U of T affiliates.

Going forward, the university aims to be a global leader in pandemic response. It has launched a new Institute for Pandemics, one of the world's first academic centers dedicated exclusively to pandemic prevention, preparation and management. <u>David Fisman has been selected to lead the division responsible for mathematical modelling</u>, as well as the development of preventative measures and strategies to reduce risk.

Canadian Institutes of Health Research: Dereliction of Duty

In the fall of 2021, Canadian provinces imposed vaccine passport systems, barring the unvaccinated from numerous social and recreational venues including restaurants, gyms, sporting events, concerts, convention centers and more. During this same period, the Canadian federal government imposed vaccine mandates for federally regulated employees and enacted a policy banning unvaccinated travellers over the age of 12 from boarding a plane or passenger train in Canada. Admittedly, the purpose of these measures was, first and foremost, to increase COVID-19 vaccine uptake. Indeed, federal policy makers had made the deliberate decision not to grant exemptions for travel on compassionate grounds in order to coerce more Canadians to get vaccinated.[10] But increasing drug use amongst the population is not, in and of itself, a reasonable justification for drastic and unprecedented measures.

The purported effectiveness of the various COVID-19 vaccines in reducing viral transmission has played a key role in the social justification for vaccine policies and restrictions. However, the clinical trials were not designed to evaluate the vaccines' ability to curtail transmission and the Omicron wave in the winter months of 2022 proved the vaccines to be ineffective at doing so. Not only was this problematic in justifying the reasonableness of limiting Charter rights and freedoms, but it called into question the "reasonable justification or excuse" for coercing vaccine uptake.

Consider the following excerpt under Section 346 of the Criminal Code:

> Criminal Code 346 (1) Every one commits extortion who, **without reasonable justification or excuse** and with intent to obtain anything, by threats, accusations, menaces or violence induces or attempts to induce any person, whether or not he is the person threatened, accused or menaced or to whom violence is shown, to do anything or cause anything to be done.

In other words, using threats, intimidation or coercive tactics without reasonable justification or excuse to interfere with somebody's freedom of choice is a serious offence under Canadian Law.

Certainly, after the Omicron surge, provinces felt they could no longer justify the use of vaccine passports and, as such, abandoned them. The federal government, however, clung to their coercive policies long after the vaccines were shown to be ineffective in curtailing community transmission. Then, along came the faux Fisman study gifting the Trudeau government what reality could not — support for their forceful actions against the unvaccinated. The Liberal government was quick to jump on the opportunity, citing the study as scientific justification for their harsh policies.

The Canadian Institutes of Health Research (CIHR) funded the Fisman study. CIHR is Canada's federal funding agency for health research; it is accountable to Parliament through the Minister of Health. The fraudulent study was cited in Parliament by the Parliamentary Secretary to the Minister of Health as justification for retaining travel restrictions against the unvaccinated. I informed CIHR of the transgression, provided solid proof and substantiation, and I asked that they set the record straight. The Agencies Presidents voted against my request.

In short, the Government of Canada funded a fraudulent study that was subsequently used to provide justification for its coercive measures at a time when there appeared to be no real justification.

That exchange demonstrates a potential means of circumventing the law. If such action goes without consequence, it opens the door to abuse either by a government in need of "science" or by researchers more interested in activism than objective research. Either way, it heightens the potential for fraudulent scientific research to be used as a tool for extortion.

Outreach: The Anti-Rackets Branch of the Ontario Provincial Police

Having exhausted the usual avenues for dealing with research misconduct and having uncovered what looked to be a greater web of malfeasance, I turned to the Ontario Provincial Police (OPP). More specifically, I reached out to the Anti-Rackets Branch of the OPP since they are experts at investigating fraud. Moreover, they have the necessary resources and capabilities at their disposal.

After spending several months detailing the case and documenting my communications with the institutions, I submitted a 150 page report and accompanying letter to OPP Commissioner Thomas W. B. Carrique. A copy was also couriered to Ontario Premier Ford's office along with a letter requesting that he support an OPP investigation. A couple of months later, I was contacted by an OPP detective for a phone interview. While the implications of the OPP's response are discussed later on, it suffices to say that a new, unorthodox approach is needed to safeguard Canadians against such malfeasance.

My efforts to have the fraudulent study corrected and researchers investigated are shown in Figure 1. The full suite of letters and correspondences with CMAJ, U of T, and CIHR are provided in the supplementary reference, *Fisman's Fraud: The Accomplices*. That, along with the OPP's take on the situation, provides a good indication of the type of response one is likely to receive when attempting to seek accountability and protections through official channels. But maybe, just maybe, Fisman's Fraud is the Establishment's Achilles heel.

Politics & Protections: The Weak Link

It is clear that individuals who chose to forgo COVID-19 vaccination have been subjected to extreme animosity and discrimination without due justification. In the case of Fisman's study, he and his two colleagues were willing to commit fraud to scapegoat the unvaccinated for product failure. Though Fisman's faux study sets a new low in research ethics and integrity, it did not occur out of the blue. It followed a series of system-wide failures that were exploited during the pandemic. The abandonment of fundamental practices in science, health care, democratic governance and law have led to the collapse of long-established safeguards to protect the health, well-being and civil liberties of Canadians. The results have been devastating.

The remainder of this book takes a look at the man and the lies behind the faux study and how his so-called science fits into the larger agenda. It concludes with a brief discussion of key safeguard failures triggered by the pandemic that have led to a cascade of reduced protections against pharmaceutical harms. A look beyond the obvious scapegoating and cheers for government overreach reveals the much larger target of Fisman's government-funded faux science: the dismantling of our last line of defense — the right to bodily autonomy.

The Fisman study is a weak link in the chain of pandemic malfeasance. That chain needs to be broken and protections put in place.

CHAPTER 3

Who is this Fisman, Anyway?

"Political ideology can corrupt the mind, and science."
— E. O. Wilson, American Scientist (1929–2021)

Canadian epidemiologist David N. Fisman has been recognized as a leader in shaping the nation's pandemic response. In January 2021, Fisman was listed amongst Maclean's power list of "50 Canadians who are breaking ground, leading the debate and shaping how we think and live."[11] While most top spots went to individuals involved in politics, business, activism and government, Fisman earned top mention in the science category for his "forceful voice demanding action" during the pandemic.

Fisman's strong and far-reaching connections have allowed him to leverage his fraudulent research to a much greater extent than is typical for scientists. He was actively involved in pandemic response at all levels of government —municipal, provincial and federal. He served on advisory councils for unions and schools and was a prominent voice that pushed for school closures and other overly restrictive measures. He has influenced court proceedings, not only via expert testimony but indirectly through his disreputable attacks on fellow scientists.

David Fisman has shown himself to be prone to hyperbole when alerting policy makers and the public on the threat of COVID-19: "We have a tsunami of death coming" he tweeted in January of 2021 as he opposed the return to in-class learning in Ontario. As described later in this chapter, his predictions could not have been farther from the truth. Such alarmism was not uncharacteristic for Fisman.

Education & Background

At the time of the COVID-19 outbreak, Fisman was a tenured professor and the Head of the Division of Epidemiology at University of Toronto's Dalla Lana School of Public Health (DLSPH).[12] He also served as a practicing physician and consultant in infectious diseases within the University Health Network and Toronto East Health Network, and was a partner at the National Collaborating Centre for Infectious Diseases (NCCID).[13]

Fisman completed his Doctor of Medicine (MD) at the University of Western Ontario and completed a residency in internal medicine at both McGill and Brown Universities. He went on to complete a fellowship at the Beth Israel Deaconess Medical Centre in Boston and received a Masters of Public Health from Harvard School of Public Health.[14] Fisman has participated in presentations and publications for the Institute on Science for Global Policy as well as the Ontario Medical Association (OMA) Speaker's Bureau where he is a member;[15] presentations generally relate to topics on infectious diseases including the connection between climate change and infectious diseases.

Early Days of the Pandemic

David Fisman caught the attention of federal Members of Parliament (MPs) early in the pandemic. In February 2020, Fisman and his colleagues were awarded a federal grant to forecast the near-term course of COVID-19 using mathematical and statistical modelling.[16] A couple of months later, May of 2020, he was invited to speak before the House of Commons Standing Committee on Health to discuss his insights into the government's response to the COVID-19 outbreak.[17]

At the meeting, Fisman acknowledged how his team's modelling work had already been influencing public policy:

I've had the gratifying experience of watching our modelling work influence policy.

—Fisman, House of Commons, May 2020

By that time, Fisman's predictions regarding the first wave had already been shown to be well off the mark — he had anticipated that Canada would see an "explosion" of cases and deaths much like Italy.[18] Far from owning up to the inadequacies of the models he helped develop, he boasted their worth. The fact that the explosion hadn't come to fruition was not a reflection of his modelling efforts, he proclaimed, but an indication of how effective the government's interventions must have been to have averted such disaster:

Make no mistake, our failure to experience these tragedies does not mean that models were wrong… Our fundamental deliverable is the non-occurrence of events.

—Fisman, House of Commons, May 2020

That is, the more inflated the COVID-19 casualty predictions were shown to be, the more successful the government's preventative actions must have been!

The MPs appeared to be quite taken by Fisman's words and the notion of made-up success. They seemed eager to hear him out, granting Fisman more than double the speaking time as other invitees at the meeting. One Liberal MP, Darren Fisher, shrugged off Fisman's failed earlier predictions remarking that "hindsight is 20/20" before giving the floor back to Fisman so he could make excuses as to why the "best advice one day can change and evolve so quickly the next." Fisman happily obliged. He stated that this virus was "a real trickster," that RNA viruses are prone to mutation, and he reiterated that mass mortality was avoided because of Canada's public health response. MP Fisher gave the explanation a proverbial two thumbs up: "This is excellent and very thoughtful testimony."

After simultaneously granting himself immunity from his own scientific forecasts and handing politicians a winning modelling strategy, he gifted them yet another political weapon:

The virus is a slippery foe, and it's a study in contradictions. I call it Schrödinger's coronavirus. It's dangerous and it's lethal, but it causes mild illness and even infection without symptoms.

—Fisman, House of Commons, May 2020

In essence, Fisman testified that (1) contradictions can be attributed to the nature of the virus and the evolving science, and (2) outrageous modelling can be used to justify harsh restrictions whilst demonstrating government success.

Fisman went on to discuss the "Trojan horse" that is asymptomatic and presymptomatic infections. He highlighted the need for aggressive testing and surveillance to find this invisible foe — the need "to hunt the virus." That strategy aligned well with the interests of two other witnesses who had been invited to give their insights: the founder and chief executive officer of BlueDot, a digital health company that specializes in tracking infectious disease; and, the president and chief executive officer of Dynacare testing and medical laboratory services.

A fourth expert in attendance — Dr. Richard Schabas, a retired former chief medical officer of health for Ontario — attempted to offset Fisman's double-talk by putting the pandemic into perspective. He warned that a myopic focus on one disease above all else had the potential to turn a tragedy amongst the mostly elderly into a societal crisis that disproportionately affects children, young families and blue-collar workers. He also warned that widespread testing, contact tracing and more lockdowns would ultimately fail to control the virus and result in much greater harm. Unlike their reaction to Fisman, the MPs appeared unenthusiastic about Schabas' views and his practical approach to a respiratory virus that was already well known to be of little risk to children and most working-aged individuals. A few days later when interviewed by TVO Today, Fisman said the following about Schabas:[19]

...he's well out of the mainstream at this point.... There was one MP who seemed to treat him (Schabas) seriously. But he didn't get a lot of questions, and he spent most of the hearing looking like someone standing next to the wall at the prom waiting to get asked to dance...

In contrast, Fisman felt that his message was well-received by the Members of Parliament. He went on to boast about his strong working relationships at the municipal, federal and international levels.

> *At this point, my colleagues and I have very productive working relationships with Toronto Public Health, Ottawa Public Health, Peel public health, with federal colleagues, with colleagues at the state level in the United States, with colleagues in South Korea and in other countries.*

> —*Fisman, TVO Today, May 2020*

The House of Commons meeting in the early months of the pandemic was rather prophetic — a glimpse into the government's playbook for their singular approach to the pandemic. They would abandon a holistic strategy and attempt to control the virus through testing and forceful government intervention. Fisman's modelling would lead the way. Dissenters would be sidelined.

Within weeks of the House of Commons meeting, two research teams listing David Fisman as a co-investigator were awarded federal funds of approximately $1 million each to measure COVID-19 incidence rates, track exposure, and study transmission and immunity dynamics.[20]

Box 2: "Paradox of Prevention"

According to Fisman's testimony for the House of Commons in May 2020, the government did such a good job in preventing widespread infection, it left Canada vulnerable to future epidemic waves because Canadians didn't build up immunity. He referred to this phenomenon as the "paradox of prevention."

Yet, Fisman would go on to spend the next several years fighting for more lockdowns and restrictions. But why, when according to the "paradox of prevention" such actions would simply kick the pandemic down the road just to rear its ugly head later?

The Science Table & Conflicts of Interest

The Ontario COVID-19 Science Advisory Table was comprised of an influential group of scientists and medical professionals that operated from July 2020 to September 2022. It informed the Ontario government's response to the pandemic and provided information to public health, to health care professionals, and to the broader public. The table's findings were also shared with the Ministry of Health's health coordination table, various stakeholders in the government's ministries and other relevant agencies.

The main task of the Science Advisory Table was to integrate, filter and contextualize the mass amounts of scientific data in order to guide Ontario's pandemic response. While the advisory table touted itself as an independent group, it cannot be said to have been representative of the greater scientific community. The table was an initiative of the DLSPH at the University of Toronto and, rather unsurprisingly, was heavily comprised of individuals affiliated with the university. While most members (apart from the Scientific Director and the Secretariat) were not paid to serve on the table, many of the members have, like David Fisman, received federal funding related to COVID-19 research.

David Fisman was among the Science Table's most vocal members. Since the early days of the COVID-19 outbreak, Fisman had been one of the most prominent critics of the Ontario government's response to COVID-19.[21] That continued to be the case throughout Fisman's tenure on the advisory table. His criticisms often accused the Ontario government of not embracing more extreme measures, or not doing so early enough, or long enough.

Fisman's role on the table drew controversy for an apparent conflict of interest when the Toronto Sun newspaper revealed that he was paid by the Elementary Teachers' Federation of Ontario (ETFO) to argue against school reopenings while serving on the Science Table. The ETFO hired Fisman as a paid consultant to give expert testimony in a dispute between the four major education unions in Ontario (including the ETFO) and the Ontario Labour Relations board. The unions were challenging the province's plan to reopen in the fall of 2020.

> *A prominent member of Ontario's science table, which advises the government on pandemic restrictions including school closures, was paid by a teachers'*

*union for offering an argument against the government's school reopening
plans at a provincial labour board hearing.*

— *Toronto Sun, Jan 26, 2021*

In his labour board submission, Fisman claimed the 2020 fall
reopening plan would "cause illness and deaths" despite zero deaths of
school-aged children caused by COVID-19 in Ontario at the time. His
submission did not mention potential harms to kids from keeping schools
closed. Later, in a January 2021 ETFO release opposing the return to in-
class learning, Fisman was the sole expert quoted to support their
argument.[22] At the time, Fisman stated that "we have to assume that there
is a lot of asymptomatic COVID-19 in schools"[23] and he took to social media
warning about a "tsunami of deaths coming" — yet another exaggerated
projection that failed to materialize.

After the conflict was first reported by the Toronto Sun, the Science
Table updated Fisman's declaration of interest form on its website to
include his involvement with the ETFO. However, Fisman had numerous
other affiliations that called into question potential conflicts of interest.
Most notably, he had also received honorariums for advisory roles from
Pfizer, AstraZeneca, the Ontario Nurses' Association, Klick Health,
JPMorgan Chase, Farallon Capital, the Canada Pension Plan, and the
infamous WE Charity, all related to COVID-19. Fisman was also paid to
participate in roundtable discussions on COVID-19 vaccines for Seqirus, a
global influenza vaccine company.[24]

In August 2021, just days after the federal election was announced,
Fisman publicly resigned from the Science Table after accusing the group of
withholding modelling data that projected a "grim fall." Whether the data
had been his conjuring or someone else's was not specified. That said, the
table's scientific director refuted the claim, spoke of the need for scientific
rigour and the inappropriateness of releasing premature estimates.[25]

Fisman again took to social media, posting his letter of resignation on
Twitter. He alleged that politics was influencing the table's final
recommendations and its decision not to share the grim projections. The
story was enthusiastically covered by legacy media; it was the top story
on the CBC (Canadian Broadcasting Corporation, a Crown corporation).
Fisman's decision to resign was praised for being neutral and non-
partisan.[26] Opposition parties were quick to attack Premier Ford for the

resignation and to demand the premier "immediately address" Fisman's allegations.[27]

Politics and hypocrisy often go hand in hand, and this exchange was no different. Indeed, Fisman appeared to have no qualms about himself playing politics with the Science Table agenda at the time.

> *Vaccine passports are a political winner in Canada. Overwhelming support, and many say they'd be more likely to use businesses if other clients were vaccinated …*
>
> — *David Fisman, July 16, 2021 (Twitter)*

> *Fourth pandemic wave in Ontario is driven by unvaccinated young adults. Vaccine passports now, please.*
>
> — *David Fisman, August 20, 2021 (Twitter)*

When tweeting about vaccine passports being a "political winner," Fisman was sure to tag Liberal MP Chrystia Freeland, Canada's Deputy Prime Minister. Apparently, the Liberal government agreed with Fisman's political assessment; vaccine mandates and restrictions became the central issue in the snap election they called just a few weeks later. Ontario Premier Doug Ford, however, had been voicing discomfort with the notion of a segregated society.

Fisman was sure to tag the Ontario premier as well as all three provincial opposition leaders in his subsequent tweet that blamed young adults for the fourth wave just ahead of the 2021/22 school year. The next day, Fisman followed up with his tweet about "grim fall" projections and two days after that he resigned from the Ontario Science Table while accusing his colleagues of political pandering. A week later, Premier Ford would succumb to mounting political pressures and flip his stance on vaccine passports.

After his departure from the table, Fisman continued to advocate his extreme views on social media, stating he found that to be more effective than going through official channels.[28]

Political & Ideological Motivations

Admittedly, Fisman had been a staunch supporter of the federal Liberals during the pandemic. In contrast, disdainful and derogatory commentary towards the provincial and federal Conservatives were commonplace on Fisman's social media feeds.[29] Throughout the pandemic, Fisman aggressively supported harsh public measures and restrictions including: lockdowns, school closures, masking in schools, vaccine mandates and travel restrictions. While both the federal Liberal government and the Ontario Conservative government had imposed stringent restrictions, Fisman often criticized the province for not going far enough.

Following his departure from the Ontario Science Table, Fisman continued to publicly berate and insult the Ontario Conservative Party while actively promoting the provincial Liberal and NDP parties and their strong vaccine mandate platforms. Leading up to the 2021 federal election and the 2022 Ontario provincial election, Fisman launched aggressive social media attacks against the Conservative parties. During the federal election campaign and within days of his resignation from the Science Table, Fisman suggested the Conservatives were promoting Nazism via coded messages.[30] Meanwhile, he was openly supporting the Liberal's calls for the segregation and exclusion of unvaccinated individuals from much of society.

In the early months of 2022, with the rise of the Omicron variant, the federal Liberal government was under increased scrutiny regarding the lack of scientific justification for their discriminatory policies. A grassroots movement protesting the vaccine mandates and restrictions had arrived on the steps of Parliament, and several lawsuits had been filed challenging the government's travel restrictions. The Prime Minister was in desperate need of scientific backing. Months earlier, before the vaccine mandates for travel had come into effect, health officials had scrambled to find any justification for the restrictions. However, emails issued by Aaron McCrorie, the Associate Assistant Deputy Minister, Safety and Security at Transport Canada, indicated that the search for such supportive evidence had come up empty.[31] Nonetheless, Trudeau doubled down on the harsh measures and ramped up his divisive rhetoric against those who refused to take the COVID-19 vaccines.

During this same period, early 2022, Fisman and his two colleagues were incorporating feedback from CMAJ into their study. As detailed in

Chapters 6 through 8, much of the rhetoric and unfounded accusations levelled against the unvaccinated by the Prime Minister appeared in the final version of the research paper. Given the need for scientific evidence, Fisman's fraudulent paper claiming that the unvaccinated put others at greater risk appears to have been rather timely. One is left to wonder whether the Fisman paper, funded by CIHR, was meant to fill the evidentiary gap.

The shoddy study quickly found its way into the hands of a Liberal MP who used it to stave off calls from opposition parties that were demanding an end to the unscientific mandates. Corporate media did their part to prop-up the Liberal-friendly study, bullhorning the faux results nationwide.

The statement of competing interests in the CMAJ publication once again called into question Fisman's many incompatible involvements. The associations listed were similar to those declared during his tenure on the Science Table. They included having served on various advisory boards related to influenza and SARS-CoV-2 vaccines for several pharmaceutical companies. He had also served as a legal expert on issues related to COVID-19 epidemiology for the Elementary Teachers Federation of Ontario (ETFO) and the Registered Nurses Association of Ontario (RNAO). In the summer of 2021, both the ETFO and RNAO had called on the Ford government to impose mandatory COVID-19 vaccination policies.[32]

The overt bias and fraudulent claims made in the CMAJ publication aligned with Fisman's political ideology, served to directly benefit the pharmaceutical companies to which he is affiliated, and, furthered the advocacy of public policy measures endorsed by the unions and associations to which he is linked. Amongst Fisman's political allies, his work has been valued as "an essential weapon" during the COVID-19 pandemic (Figure 2).

Fisman's alliances weren't the only potential conflicts of interests in the CMAJ publication. The Canadian Medical Association (CMA) and several top editors within CMAJ had also called for COVID-19 vaccinations to be made mandatory for health care workers prior to the study.[33]

Bias, whether intentional or unintentional, can manifest in many ways including: how research questions are framed; which research methodologies are used; the development (or absence) of research hypotheses; how data are selected or omitted; the statistical analysis (or lack thereof); the presentation and interpretation of the results; and, decisions regarding what to publish and where to publish the research and results.[34] The CMAJ study by Fisman, Tuite and Amoako demonstrated extreme bias in all these areas (as discussed throughout this book and provided in more detail in the supplementary guide).

Figure 2: Liberal MP Chrystia Freeland (Deputy PM & Minister of Finance) tweets support of Fisman following the ETFO conflict of interest story

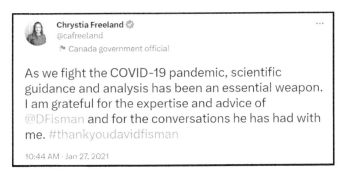

Chrystia Freeland ✓
@cafreeland
⚑ Canada government official

As we fight the COVID-19 pandemic, scientific guidance and analysis has been an essential weapon. I am grateful for the expertise and advice of @DFisman and for the conversations he has had with me. #thankyoudavidfisman

10:44 AM · Jan 27, 2021

Future Influence – Institute for Pandemics

The University of Toronto, CIHR and CMAJ are all well aware of Fisman's conflicts of interest and fraudulent research as detailed in the supporting material that was sent to each of them and to which they all acknowledged receipt. Despite this, the University of Toronto has chosen David Fisman to lead the Centre for Pandemic Readiness, one of three research centers in the newly created Institute for Pandemics (IFP) based at the Dalla Lana School of Public Health.[35]

The Centre for Pandemic Readiness is dedicated to the prevention of the next pandemic and how to limit transmission. That is, despite his precedent-setting hate science where he sought to defraud millions of Canadians of basic rights and freedoms, the University of Toronto has rewarded Fisman with a promotion to lead a new centre dedicated to research in the very area he committed the fraud. One of the co-authors of the fraudulent study, Dr. Ashleigh Tuite, will be contributing her expertise to this new enterprise as well. According to the IFP website:

The centre will perform modelling and forecasting that advises on the implications of a disease outbreak, its surveillance, transmission, case management, risk factors, protocols and response. It will also look at the impact on health system capacity and resources, as well as novel disease emergence.

It appears that the researchers who provided harmful advice during the COVID-19 pandemic will be leading the way in managing and advising on future pandemic responses.

The University of Toronto's Joint Centre for Bioethics (JCB) will also play a role in the new IFP, providing its ethical decision-making capabilities, which have helped guide responses during the COVID-19 pandemic. According to its website, partnerships are at the core of the JCB:

We partner and collaborate with government, health institutions, professional bodies, community groups, and other organizations to strengthen ethical decision-making for more positive local and global health outcomes.

Indeed, throughout the pandemic the JCB had been called upon by both the Ontario Ministry of Health and Health Canada to provide ethics input and guidance to support decision-making. The JCB Ontario COVID-19 Bioethics Table worked closely with the Ontario COVID-19 Science Advisory Table; both tables were created in 2020 with the University of Toronto taking a leading role.

But where was the Bioethics Table when Fisman's many conflicts of interest came to light? Or when the hate-fuelled and fraudulent CMAJ study was flaunted throughout the country? While the University claims it takes allegations of misconduct seriously and expects the highest standards of ethical conduct of its members, when presented with a solid complaint and irrefutable evidence of scientific misconduct and research fraud against the three authors, no investigation was undertaken. The university closed the file without addressing a single concern. Worse, the main offenders now appear to have been rewarded with even more influence in the years to come.

Fisman & U of T: Central Figures in the Pandemic

A cursory look into David Fisman's connections and influence uncovers a disturbing web, rife in conflict of interest (see Figure 3). Indeed, while tethered to numerous pharmaceutical companies and dabbling in COVID-related legal proceedings, David Fisman appears to have been a central figure in Ontario's pandemic response — an influence that extended nationally. It's little wonder Fisman made it onto Maclean's 2021 power list of influential Canadians.

One would expect that research institutes have policies and procedures in place to handle conflicts of interest that keep researchers in check. Indeed, the University of Toronto has a designated Research Oversight & Compliance Office that is dedicated to research integrity, ethics and compliance. According to its Statement on Research Integrity, the university expects its members to conduct themselves professionally and to perform and communicate their research honestly and rigorously.[36] This includes the accurate presentation and interpretation of data and factual information.

The university's integrity framework lays out the process for investigating research misconduct. Fraud, including fabrication and falsification of data and results, is explicitly mentioned in their handbook — indeed it is the very first example of research misconduct listed and deemed worthy of investigation. Willfully misrepresenting and misinterpreting findings is yet another activity the university lists as serious misconduct. The university was provided solid evidence in support of these allegations of misconduct and was alerted to the outpouring of criticisms the study had garnered from dozens of other researchers, scientists and medical professionals across Canada and abroad. Instead of standing by their core convictions on research integrity, the university chose not to investigate and not to seek remedial action.

One does not have to look far to find potential conflicts of interest at the university level which may have had some bearing on the university's decision not to investigate the overt fraud. As previously mentioned, the university had received significant funding from the federal government towards efforts to increase COVID-19 vaccine acceptance and uptake. Moreover, just weeks before Fisman et al.'s fraudulent paper was published, the university announced a major partnership with Moderna to advance the same technology that was used in the COVID-19 vaccines.

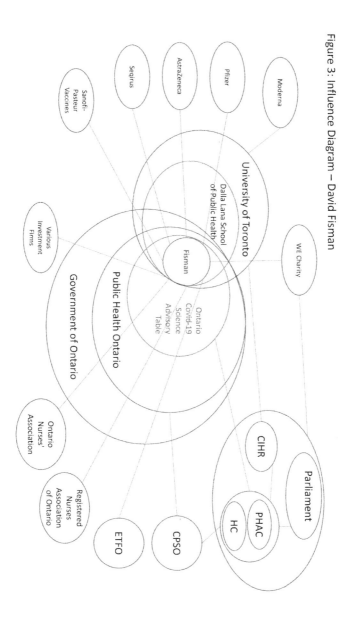

Figure 3: Influence Diagram – David Fisman

The university's vested interest in the government's vaccine policies not only calls into question their decision to turn a blind eye to the research trio's blatant misconduct, it casts suspicion on any COVID-19 vaccine-related activities undertaken by the institution. Some may even question the motivation behind the formation of the COVID-19 Science Advisory Table and its recruitment of a large number of U of T members. The table's stated purpose — to inform, and hence influence, Ontario's pandemic response, which includes advice on vaccine mandates and restrictions — raises conflict of interest concerns. In order to stave off such criticism, it is crucial that any recommendations put forth by the table follow from rigorous and scientifically sound analysis that is able to withstand scrutiny. Unfortunately, that has not been the case.

In the summer of 2021, the rollout of the COVID-19 vaccines in Canada was in full swing with the majority of Canadians rolling up their sleeves for a second dose. However, breakthrough cases had already become commonplace and by July 2021 there were serious doubts about the vaccine's ability to curb transmission. Several high-profile outbreaks amongst mainly vaccinated venues in the USA and a COVID-19 resurgence in Israel were making headlines here in Canada.

Despite the mounting warnings of potential vaccine failure, the Ontario Science Table encouraged the use of provincial "vaccine certificates" limiting entry into certain indoor venues to only the vaccinated.[37] While the table admitted there was no scientific evidence that certificates would curb transmission and that implementing such a system had serious ethical implications, they stressed the utility of passports and the obligation of governments to take the lead in developing them. The table emphasized that establishing the vaccine certificate/ passport infrastructure would make it easier to implement current public health restrictions as well as future ones. They also noted that vaccine certificates had been used in some jurisdictions to incentivize COVID-19 vaccination.

At the time, Premier Ford had voiced his objections to a vaccine passport system that would create a "split" society.

> *The answer is no. We aren't going to do it [vaccine passports]. We aren't going to have a split society.*
>
> — *Ontario Premier Doug Ford, July 15, 2021*[38]

I just don't believe in forcing anyone to get a vaccination that doesn't want it.

— *Ontario Premier Doug Ford, July 26, 2021*[39]

Just weeks later, the Ontario Premier would do a complete flip-flop. Following advice from the Science Table and a campaign pledge by the federal Liberal government to pay for the development and rollout of provincial vaccine passport systems, Ontario ushered in a two-tiered society.

Vaccinations will be mandatory for certain indoor settings where the risk of transmission is highest, because masks aren't always worn, including restaurants, bars, and casinos, among others. Enforcement will be led by bylaw officers…

— *Ontario Premier Doug Ford, September 1, 2021*[40]

Ontarians were given a mere three weeks to prepare for the segregation. On September 22, 2021 Ontario became a "show me your papers" society.

By October 2021, the month the federal vaccine mandate came into effect, the Science Table had become more aggressive in its tone regarding vaccine recommendations. The table now claimed to have "conclusive evidence" that the COVID-19 vaccines were "highly effective and safe" and that fully vaccinated individuals were less likely to transmit the virus.[41] Without producing any such proof, the table recommended that a vaccine mandate be put in place for health care workers, boldly asserting that such a policy was evidence-based. If implemented, the mandate would no longer allow unvaccinated employees to remain on the job by participating in a regular testing program.[42]

Far from presenting an objective and balanced view, the table offered up a selection of cherry-picked articles that lent support to their perspective with no acknowledgment of any controversy, waning immunity or the troubling safety signals that had surfaced, including: risk of myocarditis/pericarditis, blood clotting, neurological disorders, among many others. Even worse, the Science Table falsely stated that COVID-19 vaccines had been administered with careful monitoring and that the risks of serious side effects from the vaccines were "vanishingly low." As touched on later in Chapter 12, Canada and other countries have relied mostly on passive tracking of adverse vaccine events that captures only a very small percentage of such incidents. Even so, there have been striking safety signals.

Overall, the table angled their letter to the premier to push an agenda — mandating vaccines — with no accounting of the grave consequences that such a policy would inflict on employees. The table took no account of uncertainty whatsoever, they underplayed the risk associated with mandating COVID-19 vaccination and overplayed the benefits. In the months that followed, their assertions regarding reduced transmission benefits proved to be completely erroneous. We can only hope their comments regarding vaccine safety aren't as wildly off.

While Premier Ford ultimately rejected the recommendation to mandate the vaccine to health care workers, several Ontario hospitals and municipalities have pointed to the Science Table's endorsement as justification to impose vaccine mandates on their employees. Moreover, Peter Jüni, the paid scientific director of the table from its inception in 2020 to May 2022, provided paid testimony backing vaccine mandates in several legal proceedings.[43] A review of his expert testimony uncovers a plethora of unsubstantiated personal opinions alongside generalized statistics void of the context and detail required to make informed decisions and proper recommendations.[44] For example, it was well known that **key COVID-19 trends were dominated by the very elderly who have little to no workforce attachment.** Yet, Jüni's expert testimony and the Science Table brief that advocated for vaccine mandates relied upon dubious, population-level estimates of reduced risk associated with vaccination. Such an account is highly misleading. Certainly, it is inappropriate, if not reckless, to base far-reaching workplace recommendations on trends driven by the 70+ age group.

In summary, the Ontario Science Table had a propensity for producing overinflated projections of COVID-19 hospitalizations and ICU admittance, erring on the side of harsh restrictions and encouraging vaccine uptake even amongst groups with extremely low risk of serious COVID-19 such as children and youth.[45] Upon announcement of the table's dissolution, the Toronto Sun published an article discussing the table's "long track record of failure," highlighting several embarrassing examples of such.

The Science Table was a self-appointed and self-important group that inserted itself into Ontario's policy making early in the pandemic by putting forward modelling and projections on COVID. Despite being put on a pedestal by much of the media, the Science Table quickly proved themselves to be an organization that couldn't get basic things right.

— *Brian Lilley, Toronto Sun (Aug 26, 2022)*[46]

The bottom line is, the university had strong ties to the pharmaceutical industry as well as federal funding aimed at increased vaccine uptake. The university exerted strong influence in the community and it stood to benefit from the Science Table's questionable recommendations and the coercive vaccination tactics Fisman advocated in his fraudulent paper. Certainly, it would have been bad publicity to acknowledge that the trends touted in the paper were in fact opposite reality. But the university didn't just refuse to investigate the fraud, they ignored it altogether and went on to reinstate a discriminatory policy supported by the false findings of the Fisman study.

More specifically, in July 2022 the University of Toronto announced that it was reinstating and enhancing vaccination requirements for students and employees living in residences for the fall — mandating at least *three* doses of a COVID-19 vaccine — despite the knowledge that official government data did not support such segregationist measures.[47] The university also warned that the general vaccine requirement to attend campus was merely paused:

Vaccination requirements may be reinstated with little notice, which could result in de-enrolment or ineligibility to work.

The university's announcement came just weeks after Ontario's Chief Medical Officer of Health, Dr. Kieran Moore, held a press conference calling for a personal risk-based approach to vaccination. Dr. Moore acknowledged that the risk of myocarditis for young, healthy adults following vaccination should be weighed against the "very, very low" benefit from the COVID-19 "therapeutics."[48]

Rather incredulously, Dr. Fahad Razak, assistant professor at U of T and the (new) scientific director of the Science Advisory Table at the time, demonstrated a brazen disregard for the advice given by Ontario's Chief Medical Officer of Health. He encouraged other universities to get on board with U of T by reinstating their own vaccine mandates.[49] This direction was provided without scientific justification and ignored important studies warning of serious vaccine harm,[50] including cardiovascular damage,[51] especially among young adults.[52] Two weeks later, Premier Ford announced the dissolution of the Ontario COVID-19 Science Advisory Table.

The university's strong and unwavering endorsement of vaccine mandates and restrictions, even in the face of growing safety concerns and highly questionable effectiveness, raises serious concerns about their objectivity and ethics.

Fisman's Fraud: Life-support for a Failed Narrative

It should be noted that even when the Science Table recommended COVID-19 vaccine certificates in the summer of 2021, their science brief acknowledged that there was *"no scientific evidence of the direct impact of vaccine certificates on SARS-CoV-2 transmission."*[53] Instead, they speculated that limiting participation in certain activities to vaccinated individuals should *theoretically* reduce the risk of transmission and infection for both the vaccinated and unvaccinated. It is also worth noting that while the science brief appeared to be supportive of vaccine certificates and discussed the practical benefit of them, it fell short of directly stating they were recommended — although media coverage indicated that such was the case. The admission of there being a lack of evidence to back the table's advice is the kind of caveat that some may believe provides cover against allegations of fraud. While it can be argued that the table's support was ill-advised and potentially negligent, the disclaimer that their support was based on a "theoretical" benefit as opposed to direct evidence offers a (small) degree of plausible deniability regarding dishonesty. Importantly, this is not the case with Fisman's claims; he stated his fabricated findings as fact and, to make matters worse, he did so when there was solid evidence to the contrary. There is absolutely no ambiguity that his claims were dishonest.

It is also important to note that the Pfizer/BioNTech and Moderna clinical trials did not evaluate the vaccines' ability to reduce transmission. While the clinical trials indicated that the vaccines were effective in preventing symptomatic COVID-19 in the short-term for the Wuhan strain, it was not known if the vaccines protected against asymptomatic infection, nor had their impact on viral transmission been established. That is, when the vaccines were approved for interim use, there was <u>no evidence that the vaccines prevented transmission</u> of SARS-CoV-2 from person to person. Moreover, <u>the clinical trial reports openly stated that transmission was beyond the scope of the study</u>.

While there had been numerous speculative assertions by media, politicians, and some researchers regarding the COVID-19 vaccines' ability to reduce transmission, the actual scientific evidence admittedly had been weak and indirect. Fisman, Tuite and Amoako, however, claimed their research <u>found</u> that unvaccinated people amplify disease transmission and that their findings gave support for <u>strong,</u> restrictive measures against those who forgo vaccination. This assertion was made following the Omicron surge — the first true test of the vaccines' impact on community transmission. The vaccines had failed miserably: with almost 80% of the eligible people in Ontario vaccinated, COVID-19 cases soared to new heights. Such reality is not good for vaccine uptake. So, the researchers overwrote history with their own simulated version, blamed transmission on the unvaccinated, passed it off as fact, used their "findings" to push the pro-vaccine narrative and sought to penalize anyone who opted out.

Unlike the suggestive, indirect claims regarding transmission that have been made by many other researchers, <u>Fisman and his colleagues made strong, direct and knowingly false statements</u> — there is no room for plausible deniability of fraud.

Such a blatant act of health-related fraud and large-scale deception is not conducted for the public good. It is not utilitarian (i.e. "greatest good for the greatest number"). It is not done to protect the health and wellbeing of Canadians, as the researchers have claimed. The ultimate goal was to increase vaccine uptake — an activity for which the main author has personal stakes — and to scapegoat a vulnerable, unprotected group of individuals for product failure. While some media outlets and top NDP and Liberal politicians, including PM Trudeau, had made similar claims about the risk posed by unvaccinated persons well before Fisman's study, the fraudulent work attempted to provide scientific justification and legitimacy to the hateful rhetoric and baseless assertions.

To illustrate, Figures 4 & 5 compare the incident cases fabricated using Fisman, Tuite and Amoako's contrived model to the actual incident cases observed in Ontario during the Omicron surge. Note that the baseline conditions used in Fisman's simulation were matched to the conditions in Ontario at the emergence of Omicron. In Fisman's reality, the epidemic wave was driven by incident cases amongst the unvaccinated, as shown in Figure 4 (taken directly from the CMAJ publication). However, the official government of Ontario data — posted on the government's website and readily available to the researchers and the public at the time — showed the opposite trend (Figure 5).

Figures 6 and 7 provide a comparison of incident rates between Fisman's simulation and real-world observations. In Fisman's fabrication, the unvaccinated incident rates were disproportionately higher than the vaccinated — again, opposite reality. Many researchers have pointed out the study's contradictions to reality (see Chapter 8 for examples).

The first true test of the vaccines' impact on community transmission occurred with the emergence of the Omicron strain in the winter of 2021/22. The results were shocking: record levels of SARS-Cov-2 infections with greater incident cases and incident rates amongst the vaccinated.

The Omicron wave should have put to rest the scapegoating and the "theoretical" reduction in transmission hypothesis — and momentum appeared to be moving in that direction with the provinces dropping their vaccine passports throughout February and March of 2022. But, somehow, Fisman's fraud breathed new life into the withering theory, perpetuating a negative stereotype (a "life preserver") that entrenched politicians, media and others continue to cling to.

Figure 4: COVID-19 Incident Cases
Fisman et al.'s Simulated (FAKE) Scenario

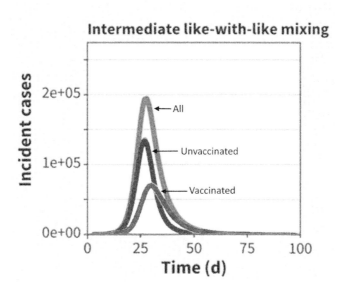

Figure 5: COVID-19 Incident Cases
Ontario (REAL) Data: (Nov. 28, 2021 - Feb. 25, 2022)

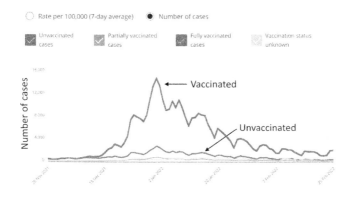

Figure 6: COVID-19 Incident Rates
Fisman et al.'s Simulated (FAKE) Scenario

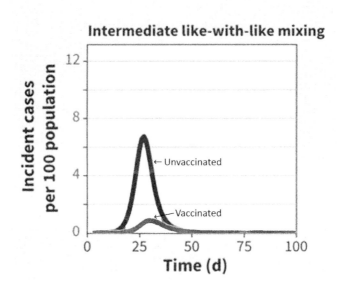

Figure 7: COVID-19 Incident Rates
Ontario (REAL) Data: Dec. 24, 2021 to Jan. 22, 2022

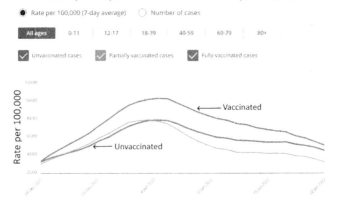

CHAPTER 4

Elements of Fraud

"There are three things in the world that deserve no mercy,
hypocrisy, fraud, and tyranny."
— *Frederick W. Robertson, English preacher (1816–1853)*

The pandemic marked an unprecedented state of societal flux. New rules and regulations were imposed, the way laws were applied and interpreted changed, and the medical sector gained greater influence in shaping public policy. This unparalleled state of uncertainty has been coupled with massive government spending with little oversight. Conditions were ripe with opportunities to conduct scientific and criminal fraud for those in a position to capitalize on this new pandemic era.

With the declaration of the COVID-19 pandemic and the ensuing state of emergency, a *massive shift* occurred in the manner in which vaccines were approved, procured, and enforced, with many of the checks and balances in the medical and legal systems suspended or abandoned altogether. Weak controls, huge financial and career incentives alongside a largely unchallenged excuse for bypassing medical and legal standards created the perfect environment for abuse. "It's a pandemic!" became the ultimate rationalization for almost any drastic measure undertaken. Opportunists made enormous gains by taking advantage of the prolonged state of emergency in ways akin to war profiteering.

Given the almost universal approach to fighting the pandemic — via newly developed pharmaceuticals — white collar crime, and in particular fraud, had the potential to impact society at levels never seen before. With demand high and money pouring out of government coffers, pharmaceutical companies and their investors stood to make fortunes. Just how much depended on how quickly they could beat competitors to the market, their ability to showcase their product as superior, and whether they could keep demand high for "updated" products to fight the latest variants.

The initial buy-in and uptake of the new genetic vaccines were astronomical. Governments bought quantities several times their population bases, securing doses well into the foreseeable future. Grand promises regarding product benefits and effectiveness were made early on and governing bodies mandated the vaccines based on those promises.

But what happens when a "miracle product" doesn't deliver?

"Science" – A Cover for Fraud

Science is a process for learning about the world, not simply a vast reservoir of knowledge to be googled and manipulated. It is not a belief, but instead hinges on testable, falsifiable hypotheses.[54] It is not a popularity contest whereby truth is contingent upon consensus or credentials. It does not censor opposing views.

When assessing scientific strength, there is a hierarchy of evidence based on objectivity, scrutiny, and uncertainty that allows one to assess the truthfulness of a theory or conjecture. To "trust the science" is to trust the scientific process, not to blindly follow the opinions of a select group of scientists or medical practitioners.

Concocting mathematical models to fabricate desired outcomes is not science. Yet, masquerading such outcomes as reality is becoming a disturbing trend. Using faux numbers to secure unfair or unlawful gain, or to swindle people out of their legal rights, isn't new. Such tactics are often exploited in the investment and medical sectors.

Analogy #1: Financial/investment fraud

Consider an investment banker who fabricates high financial returns and then tells potential investors the simulated numbers are real returns from the previous quarter. Suppose the simulation showed a huge return on investment when, in actuality, the true return was negative and investors lost money. The investment banker goes on to claim that the benefits were even greater than what he was showing because other "perks" weren't counted. The banker then attempts to persuade policy makers to impose a harsh penalty on anyone who doesn't invest in the fund. Is there any question this would be considered an egregious act of criminal fraud?

Now consider the case of David Fisman who has strong political affiliations and who has served on the advisory boards of numerous vaccine companies (as detailed in Chapter 3). Fisman, along with two of his colleagues, Afia Amoako and Ashleigh R. Tuite, concocted a faux scientific model to fabricate data that showed the unvaccinated constituted a greater risk of infection and transmission than the vaccinated, a trend *opposite* to real-world observations. They then stated the fabricated results as *fact*, made the additional claim that they likely understated the benefits of vaccination, and proceeded to use this false claim to advocate for strong actions to enhance vaccine uptake and impose harsh public health restrictions against those who declined the product.

Analogy #2: Health Care fraud

When self-serving acts of deception are committed by trusted health care professionals, whether against the health care system or patients, it affects everyone. It undermines trust in our public health institutions, impacts health care services, raises costs and taxes, and it subjects individuals to unnecessary medical procedures and risks. Below are a few relevant examples of health care fraud.

Example – Fraudulent Marketing: In 2009, Pfizer agreed to pay $2.3 billion for fraudulent marketing. Pfizer had promoted the sale of a pharmaceutical product for several uses and dosages that the US Food and Drug

Administration (FDA) specifically declined to approve due to safety concerns. Pfizer agreed to plead guilty to a felony violation for misbranding the product with the intent to defraud or mislead.[55]

Example – Fraudulent Promotion: In 2004, the Warner-Lambert company — which Pfizer acquired in 2000 — agreed to plead guilty and pay more than $430 million to resolve criminal charges and civil liabilities in connection to the illegal and fraudulent promotion of unapproved uses for one of its drug products. The company promoted the drug even when scientific studies had shown it was not effective.[56]

Example – Research Misconduct: In a December 2021 conference, the U.S. Department of Justice warned against the "dangerous consequences" of research fraud (often referred to as "research misconduct"), which serves to "undermine confidence in the health care industry as a whole."[57] From the press release:

"Scientific misconduct in clinical trials raises a number of risks, including **criminal prosecution**... The Department of Health and Human Services ("HHS"), Office of Research Integrity ("ORI") defines fraud and research misconduct as "**fabrication, falsification**, or plagiarism in proposing, performing, or reviewing research, or in reporting research results." This definition would potentially include **recording false, fabricated or misleading data, failing to disclose data that would normally be reported, submitting misleading reports** regarding the conduct of the trial, and **submitting false data** to government agencies and/or **for consideration for publication in journals**. In addition to fraud, other investigative risk areas include foreign influence, **conflicts of interests, and kickbacks**, both foreign and domestic."

Example – Falsification of Records: At the physician level, medical fraud typically involves some sort of falsification or misrepresentation of medical services or records in order to maximize payments/profit. For example: falsifying plans of treatment or medical records to justify payments; falsifying certificates of medical necessity and billing for services not medically necessary; misrepresenting diagnoses or procedures to maximize payments; misrepresenting charges or entitlements to payments in cost reports.[58]

In the current case of Dr. Fisman, Dr. Tuite and Ms. Amoako, the researchers engaged in the fabrication and falsification of data and results in order to mislead the public as well as public health officials and policy makers into believing the COVID-19 vaccines were more beneficial in reducing transmission and infection than was known to be the case.

The faux results were generated under the auspices of a public agency, submitted and published in a leading Canadian journal.

The researchers then advocated for the broad uptake of an unnecessary medical procedure — namely COVID-19 vaccination — based on their false assertions without regard for any health risks such actions would impart onto the recipients of the drugs.

What Sets This Case Apart

One might argue that during the COVID-19 pandemic, deception and misinformation ran rampant, leaving no shortage of individuals to investigate for potential acts of fraud. So why focus resources on a few mathematical modellers?

There are five main reasons why this particular case of scientific misconduct requires attention: (1) the researchers' clear intent, (2) the crucial role they played in deceiving the pubic, (3) the far-reaching impact of their fraudulent activity, (4) the willful backing by the establishment, and (5) the potential for future harm.

1. CLEAR INTENT

Often it can be challenging to establish intent; differentiating between deliberate fraud and gross incompetence can be tough. However, in the Fisman, Tuite and Amoako case, the intent is clear and provable: they outright stated their fabricated results as fact and they clearly sought to undermine the message that vaccine choice is best left to the individual. Moreover, they used their fraudulent claims to justify the infliction of harm on the unvaccinated and push for greater vaccine uptake. All the while, Fisman profited from his associations with vaccine manufacturers, and all three enjoyed perks from U of T.

2. CRUCIAL ROLE

The "follow the science" scheme requires buy-in from science "experts" who are willing to create and promote whatever material is needed to back the pro-vaccine narrative. While many scientists and medical professionals are willing to support a product they believe in, far less are willing to fabricate results in order to "fill in the gaps" or obscure an unwanted truth.

3. IMPACT

This case impacts all Canadians in multiple ways. In effect, Fisman commits fraud against everyone. Over-selling people on a drug that comes with serious risks, ignoring potential harms, and not being honest about its limitations can sway individuals to receive a treatment that provides little to no benefit to them. Some may go on to suffer serious harm as a result. Imposing restrictions on those who don't take the drug causes guaranteed harm and separates this case from all others. On a community level, the researchers' demonization of an unprotected group of individuals and the falsehood regarding the risk created for those outside the group sows societal division. It undermines trust in our research institutions. It misuses research funds and hinders the development of other, more effective courses of action and treatments.

4. WILLFUL BACKING

Individuals in key positions who were tasked with handling allegations of research misconduct backed the faux study in full knowledge of its deceitful content and scope of impact. In doing so, they demonstrated a complete disregard for academic honesty and societal well-being. The refusal of researchers and institutions to self-correct in the face of such irrefutable evidence indicates a deep-set problem that requires a system-wide review in order to determine the root cause and make the necessary changes to restore integrity.

5. FUTURE HARM

It is important to confront this fraudulent activity now, while in its infancy and manageable, before such unbridled behaviour sets a new standard and grows. Case in point, an Institute for Pandemics has already been established with Fisman set to lead the mathematical modelling efforts that will guide the nation's response to future pandemics. But mathematical simulations are not evidence — they are a playing field of what-ifs. And, if given too much influence with no accountability, mathematical modelling easily can be abused and become a tool for deception. This latter topic is discussed in Chapter 5.

It is worth emphasizing the last point — future harm. Fisman, Tuite and Amoako brought fraud to a new level within Canada, one that threatens to set a dangerous precedent going forward.

Taking Fraud to New Heights

Fisman and his co-authors engaged in fraudulent activity at three levels:

1. Scientific Fraud: Fabrication and falsification of data and results; willfully misrepresenting and misinterpreting findings in a scientific journal publication.

2. Health-related Fraud: Contriving a faux simulation to make the COVID-19 vaccines appear better than they were, to encourage greater vaccine uptake. Potential harm manifests when the fabrications influence individuals' trust in the drug which results in greater uptake, some of whom go on to suffer an adverse event.

3. *Hate Science*: Advocating harm against an identifiable[59] group of individuals (the unvaccinated) based on fraudulent claims. The researchers leveraged their positions and community standings to demonize a segment of society and attempted to defraud millions of Canadians of their fundamental rights and freedoms.

This last step represents a whole new level of degeneracy in Canada. The Fisman, Tuite and Amoako research study advocated for, and justified, inflicting harm against anyone who didn't take the COVID-19 "vaccine."

This harm was not a potential bi-product of an unintended adverse reaction to a drug. It was a direct call to strip away rights and freedoms based on fabricated results. It shows undeniable intent to injure. Sadly, the advent of this new hate science was embraced by corporate media and has contributed to extremely discriminatory behaviour and attitudes.

The fact that David Fisman is a practicing physician makes his indiscretion even more serious:

- As a physician, Fisman knows the importance of safety and efficacy in recommending pharmaceuticals, yet he bi-passed that assessment entirely. (This may be seen as negligent)

- Never mind safety, never mind effectiveness. Fisman came up with his own ill-defined nonsense measures, the "attack measure" and "blame factor", to help fabricate a narrative where he could blame the unvaccinated for infecting vaccinated people. He then aggressively proposed that individuals take the drug or face punishment. (This is construed as highly unethical)

- Fisman leveraged his position as a researcher and physician, his relationship with CIHR, and his political connections to influence public health policy for personal interests and gain. (This betrays trust)

Opportunity: Take Out the Nucleus, Collapse the Cell

Faux mathematical modelling has become the nucleus of the "follow the science" scheme.

The Omicron variant changed the playing field. Real-world data could no longer support the mass COVID-19 vaccination strategy and no amount of data manipulation could salvage it. The final tool in the "science" arsenal was to abandon reality completely and simply contrive models to support the storyline and provide the results wanted. All that was needed were willing researchers to create the faux models and lend their credentials to the cause, along with an incentivized media to propagate the findings.

By calling out the faux models and publications for what they are — fraudulent — and holding the researchers legally responsible for their activity, the scheme collapses.

The fraudulent modelling doesn't get more clear-cut than the Fisman, Tuite and Amoako case. Their actions and intent were undeniable. Their language was clear; their timing suspicious.

A strong deterrent against this activity is needed or it <u>will</u> propagate.

Fisman et al. crossed the line into overt fraud and hate science. Prosecuting the fraud provides an opportunity to expose the danger of mathematical modelling as a means of deception and its harmful impact, not only on health, but in promoting a morally degenerate society that embraces discrimination. Holding these researchers (and publishers) legally accountable would serve as a warning to all scientists tempted to commit these opportunistic crimes. Without complicit researchers like Fisman, the fraudulent "follow the science" scheme cannot be sustained.

CHAPTER 5

Replacing Scientific Fact with Fictional Simulations

"Inaccurate mathematical modeling has been frequently used throughout the COVID-19 response in order to justify lockdown measures while promoting unscientific public health edicts."
— *Ralph Behrens, MD*[60]

Throughout the pandemic there has been a dramatic shift away from solid, scientific evidence to lower quality observational data and finally to data fabrication. Whenever objective scientific evidence didn't favour the new vaccines, stakeholders looked for surrogates to take its place.

Figure 8 illustrates the slide from gathering scientific evidence to modelling fiction that has taken place over the pandemic.

Main Takeaways

CLINICAL TRIALS & EXPERIMENTAL STUDIES

When adequately designed and properly conducted using well-established scientific protocols, these studies can provide strong evidence of vaccine efficacy. These studies should be examined under a critical eye, be open, transparent, and subject to independent scrutiny. Because these studies control for confounding variables they can be used to establish causal

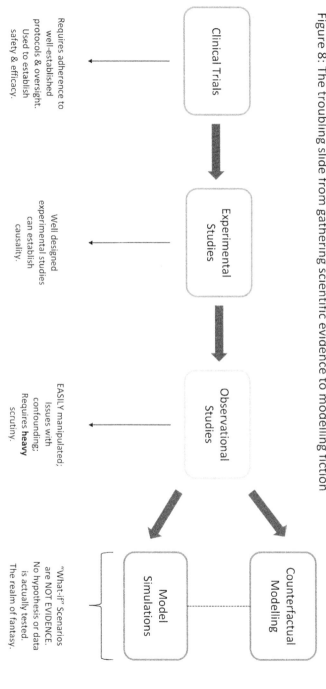

Figure 8: The troubling slide from gathering scientific evidence to modelling fiction

relationships. Such studies may also provide good evidence of vaccine safety. However, it is generally not possible to test pharmaceuticals under all possible conditions or test for all possible interactions. Thus, ongoing post-market surveillance is necessary to identify any safety signals missed during the experimental phase and to see whether products perform as well under uncontrolled, real-world conditions.

OBSERVATIONAL STUDIES

Such studies may provide supportive evidence towards a theory or hypothesis, but even when properly conducted they cannot establish cause and effect relationships on their own. The more confounding factors in a study, the easier it is to misinterpret results or manipulate the analysis. These studies require heavy scrutiny and complete transparency in order to avoid misuse. They are most useful in terms of their ability to predict an outcome. A model that fails to provide good predictions is a poor model. A researcher who routinely produces poor models is not a good statistical modeller.

COUNTERFACTUAL MODELLING

"What-if" scenarios do not provide evidence. When properly constructed they may provide a theoretical framework and insight into potential paths forward and real-world issues. Their usefulness depends on their adequacy in representing the dynamics of the system under study, whether the modelling conditions are tethered to reality and if the underlying assumptions have been scientifically validated. There is considerable latitude for misuse and rendering pure fantasy.

A more detailed discussion of how evidence and fiction factored into the pandemic response is provided in the next section. It walks through Public Health's transition over the course of the pandemic, moving away from making decisions based on hard science to increased reliance on informal logic and fictional simulations. It discusses how Fisman's study has been pivotal in this transition. The purpose of this discussion is to demonstrate that as one moves away from well-established scientific protocols and methodological rigour, the less reliable the evidence and the more room for misinterpretation and misuse. This movement is very dangerous and it is absolutely vital that it not take root. At risk is the integrity of our public health system.

While the next section provides context for the fraudulent activity, it is easy to get lost in the weeds. Statistical analysis, which forms the basis of drawing proper scientific conclusions, is heavily nuanced and is highly dependent on the competency and objectivity of the analyst — it is very easy to be bad at it. Simple designs and relationships may not be overly challenging for most researchers, but the more complex the study, the more knowledge and skill required. A poor analysis leads to erroneous conclusions, whether done purposely or not. That is why transparency and open scientific debate is crucial — to flesh out errors and expose limitations of the research.

But this case isn't about questionable data analysis or competency — the researchers didn't even use any real data. And while it can be shown that their mathematical model was of extremely low research quality (see Appendix A in the supplementary guide for a thorough critique of Fisman's study), that is also not the main issue.

At issue is that the researchers knowingly misrepresented their findings. They presented their faux results as fact in order to aggressively and unethically push pharmaceuticals for which they achieved personal gain.

The case of Fisman, Tuite and Amoako is about overt fraud masquerading as research, hoping to hide in the murky waters of scientific ambiguity. But there is nothing ambiguous about what they did.

Figure 8 illustrates Fisman et al.'s place in the hierarchy of evidence. Additional information is provided in the next section. Chapter 6 provides clear indications that politics, not science-based evidence, was the main driver behind the government's pandemic response.

Fisman vs Reality: An Exercise in Gaslighting

The main goals of an antiviral vaccine are twofold: to prevent the spread of the disease and to keep people from getting very sick and dying. Fisman et al. made strong claims about both objectives. However, the clinical trials by vaccine manufacturers were not designed to assess these endpoints and Fisman's claims didn't follow from real-world observations at the time of his study. While it was certainly hoped that the vaccines would curtail community transmission and hospitalization, these desired outcomes were never scientifically established.

Clinical Trials and Fisman's Unsubstantiated Counter Claims

Transmission: As stated in the clinical trial reports, in interviews with Pfizer executives at the time of rollout,[61] and reiterated more recently in testimony before the European Parliament,[62] the vaccines were not tested on their ability to stop transmission. Moreover, in August 2020 — months before any interim or Emergency Use authorization — immunologists were openly discussing how infection can take hold before the systemic immunity from a COVID-19 vaccine kicks in, since infection from a respiratory virus typically starts in the nose or throat.[63]

Indeed, a reduction in transmission from COVID-19 vaccination was never clinically nor scientifically established. Yet, Fisman and his two colleagues claimed that their fake simulation found that unvaccinated people were to blame for disproportionately spreading the virus.

Serious Illness & Death: Health Canada and other health agencies around the world granted interim authorization to the products based on early results from the clinical trials that indicated a significant reduction in symptomatic, clinically positive COVID-19 cases. Based on this metric, the public was informed that the vaccines were 95% effective, a figure whose meaning was widely misinterpreted.[64]

Though the vaccines appeared to greatly reduce the number of symptomatic, PCR-confirmed cases, most were mild to moderate in nature. There were very few serious COVID-19 cases in either the vaccine or placebo groups of the clinical trials. With such small numbers, the clinical trials never established a reduction in hospitalization, the use of intensive care, or even death.[65]

With assurances that the vaccines were highly effective in curtailing infection and preventing serious illness, the majority of Canadians rolled up their sleeves despite the high likelihood of discomfort in the days following the injection: fatigue, chills, fever, headaches, myalgia and injection site pain being the most common. Younger vaccine recipients (16 to 55 years of age) were more likely to experience these reactions than older vaccine recipients (more than 55 years of age) and more often after dose 2 than dose 1.[66]

Overall, a sizable proportion of individuals went on to suffer adverse events following vaccination, though mostly non-serious. However, a secondary analysis of the adverse events reported in the Pfizer and Moderna clinical trials indicates the mRNA vaccines carry an increased risk of *serious adverse events of special interest* that outweighs any risk reduction for COVID-19 hospitalization (Fraiman et al., 2022).[67] This expanding clinical body of evidence completely contradicts the assertions made in the Fisman study.

The study by Fisman et al. did not investigate the impact of vaccination on hospitalization. Yet, the researchers claimed that "unvaccinated people are creating a risk that those around them may not be able to obtain the (hospital) care they need" by disproportionately contributing to surgical backlogs. This assertion appears to be based on the researchers' misrepresentation and misinterpretation of two other studies — one a UK study and the other a USA study (i.e. of limited value to Ontario hospitalization).[68] Neither of the two studies compared the overall hospitalization rate between the vaccinated and unvaccinated groups. The incriminating assertion made by Fisman, Tuite and Amoako was inappropriate, without merit, and dangerously polarizing.

Observational Data & Fisman's Alternate Universe

In the absence of experimental data to prove the effectiveness of the vaccines in reducing transmission and hospitalization, public health agencies and others have attempted to exploit observational data ("real-world" data) to demonstrate vaccine benefit and justify aggressive vaccination campaigns. But such data is easily manipulated, there are issues with confounding factors, and results are often misreported and misinterpreted.

COVID-specific statistics such as COVID-19 cases, deaths, hospitalization and ICU occupancy depend on the definitions employed as well as testing capacity and the type of tests used — all of which have changed over time and aren't standardized across regions. Moreover, the systematic misclassification of COVID-19 cases and deaths by vaccination status — classifying cases as unvaccinated if COVID-19 positive within two-weeks following vaccination — has greatly compromised the integrity of the data and has created an inherent bias strongly favoring vaccination. In addition, COVID-19 cases, deaths and hospitalizations have been aggressively tracked whilst adverse vaccine events are passively monitored creating further bias, again favoring vaccination. As such, these measures are <u>extremely unreliable</u> indicators of the true state of emergency.

There are also issues with reporting bias. At a minimum, COVID-19 statistics should be broken down by age and the presence of any comorbid condition(s). The risk of serious COVID-19 illness and death depends greatly on an individual's underlying health issues, and risks change a thousand-fold between the oldest and youngest age groups in society. If overall statistics are given without this breakdown, there is an appearance of greater risk to the general public than is really the case, while risk to the most vulnerable is understated. Grouping data as opposed to stratifying based on key risk factors feeds into an inefficient, generalized pandemic response instead of an efficient, targeted strategy.

All too often, these kinds of reported statistics based on "real-world" data lack the necessary nuances and details required to meaningfully interpret them. Ambiguities are easily exploited to modify public behaviour and force compliance by pitting groups with different values against one another.

One may think that the above issues would be absent in Fisman's model since he doesn't use any real-world data whatsoever. Yet, many of these issues are actually amplified. Indeed, Fisman's study exploits ambiguities by not defining basic terms and conditions, thus leaving them to the readers' interpretation. For example, Fisman and his colleagues didn't even bother to define what "vaccinated" means in their model. Does it include those who are partially vaccinated with just one dose, or does it require two doses, a booster… or does "vaccinated" only refer to those who are "up-to-date"? Without knowing this, how can the outcomes be meaningfully interpreted?

Fisman, Tuite and Amoako also appear to conflate vaccine effectiveness and efficacy with immunity. These terms have separate meanings yet seem to be used interchangeably within the paper. Their model makes no use of Ontario's demographics, whatsoever, and omits key factors. A discussion of the model's main shortcomings is provided in detail in the supplementary guide (Appendix A, Concern #2: Poorly constructed, inadequate modelling). It appears the authors made no attempt to capture real-world transmission dynamics; the model basically serves as a disinformation piece.

Even when properly conducted, *observational studies cannot establish causality* ("correlation does not imply causation"). The use of COVID-19 statistics and time series data is *highly nuanced;* there are a lot of factors at play — so much so that the public has been subjected to heavily conflicting narratives depending on the agenda of the person(s) doing the study.

Researchers must be *extremely* careful when making claims based on "real-world" observational data, especially in the absence of clinical trials or experimental studies to back up the assertions. Government and public health officials from Canada and around the globe made lofty, hopeful promises, many of which fell apart under scrutiny and with the passage of time. In short, the narrative changed rapidly and so did the measures used to characterize it. This shifting of the goalposts was needed to tune and recalibrate the narrative in order to justify mass vaccination whenever real-world data could no longer be twisted to support earlier claims.

Initially people were sold on a two-dose regime with talk of attaining herd immunity through vaccination.[69] This was accompanied by strong public statements from the US Centers for Disease Control and Prevention (CDC) and others that "vaccinated people do not carry the virus and don't get sick."[70]

Soon after, however, there was evidence of breakthrough cases and the narrative shifted to "vaccines stop most transmission."[71] But by May 2021, breakthrough cases had become the norm, the CDC began tracking only breakthrough cases that lead to hospitalization and death. The narrative shifted focus to "vaccines are very effective at preventing severe disease and death."[72]

But the number of vaccinated individuals testing positive for COVID-19 continued to climb and they began taking up an increasing proportion of hospitalizations. Indeed, studies around the globe reported a steady decline in vaccine effectiveness over time, dropping from 95% down below 50% to close to zero and then dipping into the negatives.[73] Despite this devastating trend, health officials across Canada continued to recommend vaccines for the general population with the message shifting to "stay up-to-date" with your boosters as a means of combating the quickly waning immunity.

By December 2021 when the Omicron wave hit, over 81% of the total population in Canada had received a COVID-19 vaccine. COVID-19 cases and hospitalizations surged, hitting record highs. By May 2022, it was estimated that half of all Canadians may have been infected with COVID-19.[74] The Institute for Health Metrics and Evaluation (IHME) estimated that, as of December 12, 2022, 90% of people in Canada had been infected at least once.[75]

The number of daily COVID-19 cases and hospitalization in Canada since the start of the pandemic are illustrated in Figures 9 and 10, respectively. It seemed the Omicron variant pounded a stake through the heart of the vaccine narrative.

With the emergence of the Omicron variant, no amount of data manipulation could save the flailing vaccine narrative. Enter Fisman, Tuite and Amoako's reverse-world simulation: blame the small proportion of unvaccinated Canadians for the apparent vaccine failure.

Figure 9: Daily COVID-19 Cases, Canada

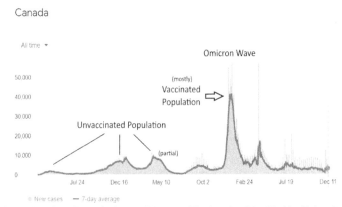

Source: Data from Center for Systems Science and Engineering, Johns Hopkins University
March 2020-Dec 2022

Figure 10: Number of COVID-19 patients in hospital, Canada

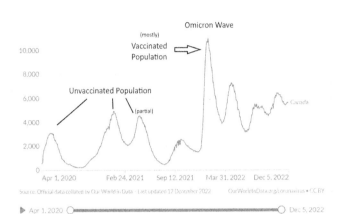

Source: Official data collated by Our World in Data – Last updated 17 December 2022   OurWorldInData.org/coronavirus • CC BY

Shortly after the publication of Fisman et al.'s fabricated results that attempted to scapegoat unvaccinated Canadians, the Public Health Agency of Canada published a counterfactual study of what-ifs to illustrate what may have happened in Canada had the vaccines and aggressive public health measures such as lockdowns not been used to control the COVID-19 epidemic.[76] Unsurprisingly, the publication, co-written by Canada's Chief Public Health Officer Theresa Tam, concluded that Canada's response was effective, though not perfect, with potentially tens of millions of cases averted, a couple million fewer hospitalizations and hundreds of thousands fewer deaths. While the model is easily shown to be self-aggrandizing nonsense with no basis in reality,[77] the important thing to understand is that:

"What-ifs" are NOT evidence. Neither counterfactual models nor simulations of the sort done by Fisman and his colleagues are evidentiary — even had they been done correctly and honestly.

No hypothesis or data is actually tested in these models. Moreover, in the case of Fisman's simulation and Tam's counterfactual exercise, there was no attempt to undertake even the most rudimentary validation exercises to ground their studies in reality. These publications demonstrate how easy it is for such modelling to completely detach from reality and enter the realm of fantasy. Unconstrained by real data or actual evidence of any kind, influential researchers and medical practitioners like Fisman and Tam are free to pass off their biases as expert testimonials and push their ideology and self-serving interests as science.

But science is rooted in testable explanations and predictions, not expert make-believe. Scientific theories are modified or replaced when new information disagrees with the current theory. In the case of COVID-19 vaccines, substantial evidence not only proves that they do not stop infection or transmission, it suggests they may do the opposite depending on time since last dose.

This shift from solid lines of evidence to contrived make-believe and, in Fisman's case, clear fraud, is dangerous. We cannot allow this to become the new standard.

CHAPTER 6
Politics & Fake Science

"In politics, stupidity is not a handicap"
— Napoleon Bonaparte, French military leader and emperor (1769–1821)

How Politics Shaped the Public Health Response

While models and predictions put forth by experts such as those on the Ontario Science Table have been habitually wrong, the politics feeding the public health messaging has been remarkably consistent. Politicians and public health officials locked into COVID-19 vaccination early on; their commitment to this never wavered, regardless of what the data indicated or how poorly the vaccines performed.

Less than a year into the pandemic, vaccines were already being touted as the way out. In November 2020, a Global News headline read: "'A big sigh of relief': Trudeau says coronavirus vaccines in spring will begin end of pandemic."[78]

> *People just need to hang on. It's not forever, it's only for a few more months.*
>
> *— Trudeau, Nov 2020*

At the time, Trudeau and Tam were bracing the public for upcoming

Christmas restrictions to help reduce spread and keep hospitals from being overfilled. Indeed, provincial restrictions were imposed prior to Christmas and then extended into late January and early February.[79] Despite Trudeau's assurances that the solution to the pandemic was at hand, clinical trials at the time had made no promise of reduced transmission nor had they established a reduction in hospitalization.

In early February, Trudeau provided an update on the COVID-19 situation and vaccine rollout to assure Canadians that things were on track:[80]

> *We all want to be done with this pandemic as soon as possible. And that's exactly why we're focused on vaccines... we will get everyone vaccinated by September.*
>
> *— Trudeau, Feb 2021*

The uptake for the first vaccine dose began ramping up in mid-March 2021 at which time COVID-19 cases also began to climb, marking the commencement of the "third wave." By early April, several provinces went into lockdown, once again, and people were encouraged to get their vaccination as a way out of the lockdown cycle.[81]

> *Provinces across Canada are entering another round of tightening restrictions and lockdowns as infection rates from more contagious variants grow. Provinces have been cycling through various states of restrictions and lockdowns since last March.*
>
> *"There is a way to break the pattern, and the way to break the pattern is through mass vaccination," Infectious disease specialist Dr. Isaac Bogoch told CTV's Your Morning.*
>
> *— CTV News, April 8th 2021[82]*

> *A "freer" and "more normal" summer might be possible this year depending on whether COVID-19 cases drop and at least 70% of Canadians get vaccinated, according to Prime Minister Justin Trudeau.*
>
> *— BIV, May 11th, 2021[83]*

About 60% of the population rolled up their sleeve for the shot in the spring of 2021 with the 70% goal for the first dose reached by early summer.

The 70% vaccination objective was echoed by leaders around the globe, the goal having been set by the World Health Organization (WHO) early in the pandemic.[84] As time went on, the goalpost for Canadians crept upwards: 70% vaccinated to 75% to 80% … to talk of mandatory vaccination with the potential for ongoing booster shots.

Recall that in May 2021, Prime Minister Justin Trudeau claimed to oppose vaccine passports, saying they would be divisive. He publicly stated the following:

> *We're not a country that makes vaccination mandatory.*

> — *Trudeau, May 2021*[85]

But during that same time, the federal government was procuring **hundreds of millions of doses** of COVID-19 vaccines,[86] enough guaranteed supply for every man woman and child to receive 3 doses in 2021, plus hundreds of millions more doses secured for 2022, 2023, 2024 — in total enough for **10 doses for every Canadian**.[87]

If no mandates or passports were on the table, why would Canada purchase such massive quantities?

If our government believed the 2-dose regiment was as effective as they were claiming, why lock Canadians in to the purchase of a couple of hundred million doses, with option to buy up to 400 million for a population of only 37 million Canadians?

Within months of Trudeau's statement, he campaigned on bringing in mandatory vaccination for federal workers and imposing travel restrictions. He also promised provincial governments $1 billion to help pay for vaccine passports.[88]

> *If you don't want to get vaccinated, that's your choice. But don't think you can get on a plane or a train beside vaccinated people and put them at risk.*

> — *Trudeau, August 2021*

At the time, there was no scientific basis for the restrictions nor the mandates, nor the accusations against those who chose not to receive injections. Indeed, mRNA vaccines were granted interim authorization without establishing reduced transmission[89] and by July 2021 there were already several reports of large-scale COVID-19 outbreaks amongst mostly vaccinated individuals. Moreover, the CDC was reporting that fully vaccinated people who get infected carry as much of the virus in their nose as unvaccinated people.[90]

One prominent outbreak stemming from Independence Day celebrations in Barnstable County reported nearly 500 COVID-19 cases amongst Massachusetts residents, 74% of whom were fully vaccinated. Five were hospitalized: one was not vaccinated and had multiple underlying medical conditions; four were fully vaccinated, two of whom had underlying medical conditions.[91] Meanwhile, Fisman was busy tweeting about the "anti-vaxxers" in full support of placing heavy restrictions on the unvaccinated so that those more deserving of freedom could get their lives back (his remarks are discussed in the next chapter).

During that same period, a resurgent COVID-19 outbreak in Israel was also making headlines across the globe.[92] Israel had led the way in COVID-19 vaccination — it was the first country to fully vaccinate the majority of its citizens, doing so by the end of March 2021, several months ahead of other countries including Canada.[93] But by mid-June there were already strong indications of waning immunity against the Delta variant of SARS-CoV-2. This reduction in effectiveness was observed across all age groups a few months after receipt of the second dose of vaccine.[94] On July 30, 2021 the Israeli Minister of Health approved the administration of a booster (3rd dose) of COVID-19 vaccine to persons who had been vaccinated at least five months previously.

Despite these early warning signs that vaccine effectiveness was much lower than the advertised 95%, the Trudeau Liberals chose to scapegoat the unvaccinated for COVID-19 transmission and to campaign on vaccine mandates. It seemed that the scientific and legal default of having to prove necessity and effectiveness had been supplanted by requiring citizens to come up with irrefutable proof that the vaccines were not safe and that they had absolutely no benefit — an absurd reversal, especially when government and pharmaceutical companies control data collection and data access.

In early September 2021, Ran Balicer, chair of the expert advisory panel to the Israeli government and chief innovation officer for the health service organization, Clalit, issued the following warning to other countries:[95]

> *"Waning immunity is a real challenge that every country needs to prepare a contingency plan to tackle."*
>
> — *Balicer, Israeli Expert Advisor, September 2021*

In the weeks that followed, instead of acknowledging the vaccines' obvious shortcomings in regards to preventing infection and transmission, provinces implemented their vaccine passport systems. Upon re-election with a minority government, Prime Minister Trudeau made good on his threats to mandate COVID-19 vaccination for the federal workforce and for federally regulated transportation sectors. Travel restrictions against the unvaccinated were imposed shortly thereafter.[96]

By early fall, the idea of waning immunity from vaccines gained traction and booster shots were being promoted and normalized in the media as "a standard part of the vaccination schedule."[97]

Then, in mid to late November 2021, Omicron emerged in South Africa and it quickly became clear that the vaccines would not be effective in curtailing the spread of the virus. By early December, before the Christmas surge, even top pharmaceutical spokespersons were casting doubt on the effectiveness of the vaccines in fighting the Omicron variant.

> *There is no world, I think, where [the effectiveness] is the same level ... we had with [the] Delta [variant]... I think it's going to be a material drop. I just don't know how much because we need to wait for the data. But all the scientists I've talked to ... are like, "This is not going to be good."*
>
> — *Stéphane Bancel, Moderna CEO*[98]

> *We must be aware that even triple-vaccinated are likely to transmit the disease...It is obvious we are far from 95 per cent effectiveness that we obtained against the initial virus.*
>
> — *Ugur Sahin, CEO of BioNTech*[99]

With about 80% of the population "fully vaccinated," Canada witnessed record-breaking highs in the number of daily COVID-19 cases over Christmas 2021. Despite the vaccines obvious failure at preventing infection and transmission, and despite the warnings from the pharmaceutical companies admitting that an additional dose of their product would not likely provide adequate protection, politicians and public health officials continued to push for vaccination and urged those "fully vaccinated" to get their booster.

As cases continued to surge, provinces accelerated their booster dose rollout and re-introduced temporary lockdown measures to help blunt transmission and prevent hospitals from becoming overwhelmed.[100] Moreover, the federal government continued to push provinces to make vaccination mandatory.

On January 7th, 2022 a CBC headline read: "Provinces could make vaccination mandatory, says federal health minister." An excerpt from the article read as follows:[101]

> Provinces are likely to introduce mandatory vaccination policies in the coming months to deal with surging COVID-19 caseloads, Health Minister Jean-Yves Duclos said today.
>
> "What we see now is that our health care system in Canada is fragile, our people are tired, and the only way that we know to get through COVID-19, this variant and any future variant, is through vaccination," Duclos said.

Days earlier, Trudeau was putting blame for the COVID-19 surge and general public restrictions on the unvaccinated, claiming that while most people had "stepped up" and got their COVID-19 shots, the unvaccinated remained a problem.

> When people are seeing cancer treatments and elective surgeries put off because beds are filled with people who chose not to get vaccinated, they're frustrated…When people see that we are in lockdowns or serious public health restrictions right now because of the risk posed to all of us by unvaccinated people, people get angry.[102]
>
> — Trudeau, January 5, 2022

At the time of these remarks, official Government of Ontario data showed that **COVID-19 incident rates amongst the vaccinated were markedly higher than those of the unvaccinated**. Indeed, even David Fisman commented on how many of his vaccinated acquaintances had COVID-19.

> *Hearing from so many 2 and 3 dose vaxxed friends and colleagues with mild covid... For the love of sanity: get vaccinated.*
>
> — *Fisman, January 5, 2022*

Recall, provinces had implemented vaccine certificates months prior to the Omicron surge and the federal government had restricted travel for the majority of unvaccinated individuals. It seemed the Omicron variant had travelled to Canada on the backs of vaccine passport holders.

Regardless of the actual facts, on January 15th, 2022 the federal government proceeded to impose further border restrictions on the unvaccinated, including quarantine requirements on Canadian truck driver's who were not fully vaccinated and denying entry to unvaccinated or partially vaccinated foreign national truck drivers.[103] This sparked border blockades at Coutts Alberta and Windsor Ontario, as well as a massive trucker convoy ("The Freedom Convoy") which arrived in Ottawa on the eve of January 28th, marking the start of a 3-week long protest.[104]

In the midst of the protest and growing evidence of the vaccines' inability to curtail transmission, provinces began relenting on mandates and scrapping their vaccine passports, beginning with Saskatchewan and Alberta. PEI, Ontario and Quebec followed suit within days.[105] By the end of February, nine of the ten provinces had announced a plan to drop their vaccine passports.[106]

Federal opposition parties (the Conservatives and the Bloc Québécois) along with several provincial premiers requested that the federal government drop its COVID-19 restrictions as well. Saskatchewan Premier Scott Moe noted that vaccination was not reducing COVID-19 transmission and aptly pointed out that both he and Prime Minister Justin Trudeau had contracted the Omicron variant, despite receiving three shots of the vaccine, including a booster shot.[107] He called for the end of the federal border policy for truckers.[108]

Because vaccination is not reducing transmission, the current federal border policy for truckers makes no sense. An unvaccinated trucker does not pose any greater transmission than a vaccinated trucker.

— *Saskatchewan Premier Scott Moe, January 29, 2022*

Days later he called on the federal government to outline a plan to remove COVID-19 mandates and restrictions.

Every province is now outlining its plan to remove mandates and restrictions. We are calling on the Trudeau government to do the same.

— *Saskatchewan Premier Scott Moe, February 9, 2022 (Twitter)*

Instead, Trudeau doubled-down on his pro-mandate rhetoric and responded to the convoy by enacting the Emergency Act — the successor to the War Measures Act — for the first time in Canadian history.[109] Canada had resorted to the prior War Measures Act only three times: World War I, World War II, and the October 1970 Front de libération du Québec (FLQ) crisis.

Under cross-examination during the Public Order Emergency Commission, Deputy Prime Minister Chrystia Freeland conceded that the true purpose of the cross-border regulations on truckers was to compel as many Canadians as possible to get vaccinated.[110]

As Ottawa declared war against the trucker convoy, Fisman took to Twitter to once again affirm his support for vaccine mandates and passports.

We now know that a full (3 dose) vaccine schedule prevents: omicron infection, omicron transmission, and serious illness from sars-2. Vaccine mandates and passports remain smart…

— *David Fisman, Feb 17, 2022 (Twitter)*

Despite his post just six weeks earlier stating that he knew so many double and triple vaccinated individuals getting COVID-19, Fisman's support for vaccination and the use of mandates remained in lock-step with that of the Trudeau government.

In the weeks that followed, real-world data continued to portray dismal protection from vaccination, with reported effectiveness of boosters in preventing symptomatic disease dropping to about 35% in just 10 weeks.[111] Indeed, as the weeks and months went on, **incident rates amongst the boosted were shown to be markedly higher than all other groups.**

By mid-March 2022, British Columbia, the last province to hold out against dropping its vaccine passports, announced that it too would do so, with the system officially ending April 8th.

PM Trudeau now stood alone, holding strong to the vaccine mandate for federal employees as well as border and travel restrictions.

On April 25th, Fisman, Tuite and Amoako's fraudulent study was published which attempted to give PM Trudeau's nonsensical mandates the appearance of scientific legitimacy. Like the PM, the researchers falsely accused the unvaccinated of putting the vaccinated at greater risk and attempted to blame the unvaccinated for the cancellation of surgeries and backlogs. On April 29th 2022, just four days after its publication, Liberal MP Adam van Koeverden cited the study in Parliament as justification for continuing the travel restrictions when "virtually no other country requires them for domestic travel for their citizens" (Conservative MP Blaine Calkins).

Six weeks later, amidst mounting pressure and an upcoming court challenge against the federally imposed travel restrictions, the Trudeau government finally announced the *suspension* of its COVID-19 vaccine requirements for domestic and outbound travel as well as the suspension of vaccine mandates for federal public servants and transportation workers. As of June 20th, 2022 the requirements were dropped with the caveat that the measures could be brought back at any time.

Federal court documents stemming from the challenge against the travel restrictions reveal that the government's travel ban decision in 2021 had not been based on science.[112] Yet, the Trudeau government imposed one of the most sustained stringent policies on domestic movement among G10 countries. Indeed, Canada experienced some of the most restrictive public health measures on the planet.[113]

Even upon suspending the harsh measures, PM Trudeau reiterated his unscientific and discriminatory stance against the unvaccinated, stating that they should accept the consequences of their decision including lost employment, restricted access to transportation, and severe lifestyle restrictions.[114]

> *It was their choice and nobody ever was going to force anyone into doing something they don't want to do. But there are consequences when you don't. You cannot choose to put at risk your co-workers. You cannot choose to put at risk the people sitting beside you on an airplane.*
>
> — *Trudeau, June 2022 CBC Radio's The House*

Within days of suspending the domestic travel restrictions, government lawyers filed a motion seeking to shut down the court challenge on the grounds that it was now moot. The judge ruled in their favour in late October 2022. The decision has been appealed with a court date scheduled for the fall of 2023.

By September 2022, there was talk of seasonal boosters to top-up waning immunity[115] and Health Canada authorized the first adapted version of the COVID-19 vaccine which targeted the original SARS-CoV-2 virus and the Omicron variant. Canadians were encouraged to take this bivalent vaccine along with the seasonal flu shot.[116]

That fall, there was also talk of combining the flu vaccines and COVID-19 vaccine into one. In fact, Moderna had already begun actively promoting a combined 3-in-1 vaccine to fight COVID-19, the seasonal flu and RSV. They were anticipating regulatory approval within a year.[117]

By the fall of 2022, some Canadians[118] had received their sixth shot and were awaiting their seventh.[119]

House of Cards

While dishonesty in politics is nothing new, most people believe in the rigours of science and trust that researchers and public health officials have their best interests at heart.

It was clear from the onset that the political agenda was to get the new genetic vaccines into the arms of every Canadian, with the option to administer top-ups for the foreseeable future. The strategy was not based on objective science, nor was it founded on solid evidence. Moreover, as new evidence emerged that revealed serious safety concerns and shortcomings in effectiveness, the government continued to recommend wide-spread uptake, often doubling down on its pro-vaccine stance.

Due to their rapid development and deployment (months instead of a decade), the scientific community and the governments they advised knew full well that a multitude of scientific unknowns would play out over time in the way of vaccine effectiveness; duration of protection (i.e. rate of decay and potential need for boosters); viral evasion of the protection; and the frequency, severity and timelines of post-vaccination adverse effects.[120] But instead of taking a strategic, measured approach and offering the vaccine to vulnerable groups who were at highest risk of serious COVID-19, Health Canada approved use for the masses. Indeed, Health Canada and top public health officials promoted the use of the vaccines to the general public without regard for individual risk-benefit assessments. **This action is contrary to their own well-established risk management decision-making framework that specifically calls for a risk-benefit approach.[121]**

It is important to note that our Public Health Agency is not an independent scientific community. The Chief Public Health Officer is appointed by the government in power. There is no doubt that during the pandemic the public health response was greatly influenced, if not driven, by political forces. Shortcuts were taken in the drug approval process and post-market surveillance, including a lack of adequate ongoing risk-benefit assessments.

Medical doctors have played a predominant role in the vaccination campaign. However, most MDs operate under the assumption that regulatory agencies have done their due diligence and that approved drugs are safe and effective. It is not their job to critically evaluate them, nor do they have time to do such a thing for every drug they administer. Moreover, most MDs are not experts in the assessment of research and scientific evidence, risk-benefit analysis, performance measurement or statistical data analysis. Much support from the medical community has been based on trust in the functional, albeit not perfect, system in place prior to the pandemic.

MDs who did not support the vaccine recommendations either remained silent or faced reprimand by the College of Physicians and Surgeons. In Ontario and throughout Canada, if an MD were to voice any opinion that called into question the safety and effectiveness of the COVID-19 vaccines, they would risk disciplinary action and possibly lose their license to practice medicine.[122] Many physicians had no choice but to take the genetic vaccines themselves to continue practicing in hospitals.

Given the political stakes, the connections between pharmaceutical companies, government and researchers, as well as the clear conflicts of interest and punitive measures imposed on opposing voices, it is important that vaccine recommendations and invasive public health measures be based on solid, objective evidence as opposed to expert opinion or a perceived consensus.

When clinical trials failed to provide evidence of reduced transmission or any other clinically relevant benefit from the vaccines (such as reduced hospitalization, serious illness or death), focus shifted to heavily biased "real-world" studies. When those also failed to support widespread vaccination efforts, politicians and public health authorities concocted counterfactual "what if" models to demonstrate that "it could have been worse" and to claim that vaccines and public health measures resulted in huge, unverifiable benefits (as discussed in the previous chapter).

Fisman, Tuite and Amoako went one step further: they concocted a model to simulate data opposite reality then attempted to pass the findings off as facts. They used their faux facts to demonize the unvaccinated and blame them for higher transmission that put the vaccinated at greater risk. They claimed their results provide strong support for imposing restrictions on the unvaccinated including the use of vaccine passports as well as punitive measures imposed by the Trudeau government.

Fraudulent modelling has become the backbone of the "follow the science" scheme. Without it, the house of cards collapses.

Checks and balances are put in place for a reason: to protect against abuse and harm. When such measures are circumvented and trust (i.e. in science) is abused, the potential for fraud is huge.

The massive uptake of genetic vaccines and mRNA technology has laid the foundation for future mRNA-based vaccines and treatments.[123] Checks and balances need to be adhered to in order to ensure health and safety is at the forefront. *We cannot allow fabricated results to masquerade as scientific evidence.*

Fisman, Tuite and Amoako committed fraud of a heinous nature which has substantially harmed a large group of individuals. If this hate science is not corrected it sets a very low bar for future research.

The next chapter provides specific examples of the fraudulent statements and defamatory remarks made by Fisman, Tuite and Amoako. The reaction of other scientists to the fraudulent study follows in Chapter 8.

CHAPTER 7

Fisman's Fraudulent Statements

"As an instance of fraud, the fabrication of data is a particularly blatant form of misconduct... Fabricating data is making it up, or faking it. Thus, it is a clear instance of a lie, a deliberate attempt to deceive others."
— *Goldfarb & Pritchard (Ethics in the Science Classroom, 2000)*[124]

Fabrication and falsification of data and results are two of the most severe violations of research integrity.

Data fabrication is the act of making up data and reporting the made-up data as a true reflection of events. An example of fabrication includes artificially creating data when it should be collected from an actual experiment or observation.[125]

Falsification involves a deliberate manipulation of the research process to produce a desired result, including leaving out data that goes against a desired result.[126]

Fisman et al. concocted a model to generate the results they wanted, completely omitting any reference to readily available real-world data that contradicted their results (falsification). They went on to state the contrived results as facts (data fabrication) and then proceeded to inform public policy based on the fabricated results. The researchers continued to push the false narrative long after numerous scientists rebuked the findings and provided evidence of the findings' falsity. This indicates a willful misrepresentation and misinterpretation of research findings.

This chapter provides an account of specific fraudulent statements contained in the Fisman et al. publication as well as a listing of some of the derogatory comments and comparisons levelled against the unvaccinated in the aftermath of the study. An examination of how the study has been used by the Trudeau government is also provided.

Knowingly Misrepresenting Material Fact

On April 25th, 2022 a misleading and factually incorrect research paper written by David Fisman and two of his colleagues, Afia Amoako and Ashleigh R. Tuite (the "authors"), was published by the Canadian Medical Association Journal (CMAJ):

> David N. Fisman, Afia Amoako, Ashleigh R. Tuite. "Impact of population mixing between vaccinated and unvaccinated subpopulations on infectious disease dynamics: implications for SARS-CoV-2 transmission." CMAJ 2022;194:E573-E580. DOI: https://doi.org/10.1503/cmaj.212105.

The highly erroneous "findings" of this Canadian paper were quickly taken up and disseminated by dozens of national and international media outlets. The paper itself contains numerous false and defamatory statements including the main "result":

> *...we found that the choices made by people who forgo vaccination contribute disproportionately to risk among those who do get vaccinated.*

The above quote, taken directly from the CMAJ paper, asserts a finding regarding choices made by people despite a complete absence of people or real-world observations in the study.

The authors go on to state their findings as fact and falsely claim that their fictitious fact supports "strong public actions" that limit the rights and freedoms of those who forgo COVID-19 vaccination. The authors acknowledge that imposing such actions based on their fiction comes at a cost to targeted individuals. The following passage is taken directly from the publication:

> *The fact that this excess contribution to risk cannot be mitigated by high like-with-like mixing undermines the assertion that vaccine choice is best left to the individual and supports strong public actions aimed at enhancing vaccine uptake and limiting access to public spaces for unvaccinated people, because risk cannot be considered "self-regarding." There is ample precedent for public health regulation that protects the wider community from acquisition of communicable diseases, even if this protection comes at a cost of individual freedom.*

Not only are the above statements entirely false, they clearly expose a group of identifiable individuals (the "unvaccinated") to psychological, financial and discriminatory harm. Some of the ways unvaccinated people have been identified or singled out include: (1) the requirement to disclose their vaccination status to employers as a condition of continued employment, (2) the requirement to disclose their vaccination status to various organizations in order to gain entry or participate in functions, and (3) being, or having been, conspicuously excluded from various aspects of daily life due to their vaccine status.

Fisman, Amoako and Tuite fabricated a fictitious result, masqueraded it as a true scientific finding, then used it to advocate restricting the fundamental rights and freedoms of millions of identifiable Canadians.

Defamatory Statements

In the days following the fraudulent CMAJ publication, the false and defamatory conclusions of the study made headlines across Canada and beyond. The following is a sample:

- *Merely hanging out with unvaccinated people puts the vaccinated at higher risk: study* by Eric Schank, *Salon. (April 27, 2022)*[127]

- *Unvaccinated People Increase Risk of Covid Infection Among Vaccinated, Study Finds* by Robert Hart, *Forbes. (April 25, 2022)*[128]

- *Unvaccinated people threaten the safety of individuals vaccinated against SARS-CoV-2* Reviewed by Emily Henderson, B.Sc., *News Medical. (April 25, 2022)*[129]

- *Unvaccinated disproportionately risk safety of those vaccinated against COVID-19, study shows* by Andrea Woo, *The Globe and Mail. (April 25, 2022)*[130]

- *Unvaccinated People Create Higher Risk for Vaccinated, Study Says* by Ralph Ellis, *WebMD. (April 27, 2022)*[131]

- *Study: Unvaccinated People Increase COVID-19 Risk, Even Among Vaccinated People Healthline. (April 25, 2022)*[132]

- *Unvaccinated people increase risk of COVID-19 infection among vaccinated: study* by Irelyne Lavery, *Global News. (April 25, 2022)*[133]

- *Mixing with the unvaccinated increases COVID-19 risk for the vaccinated, study finds* by Morgan Lowrie, *Canadian Press,*[134] *Toronto Sun,*[135] *Vancouver Sun,*[136] *Calgary Sun,*[137] *Toronto Star,*[138] *Montreal Gazette,* [139] *National Observer,*[140] *National Post,*[141] *Times Colonist, CTV News,*[142] *The Chronicle Journal,*[143] *Canoe.com,*[144] *OHS Canada,*[145] *Prince George Citizen,*[146] *The Abbotsford News,*[147] *The Williams Lake Tribune,*[148] *The Edmonton Journal,*[149] *Richmond News,*[150] *The Chilliwack Progress,*[151] *MYMcMurray.com,*[152] *Castanet.net,*[153] *(April 25, 2022)*

- *Mixing with unvaccinated increases COVID-19 risk for vaccinated: Study* by Michael Ranger, *CityNews Everywhere (April 25, 2022)*[154]

- *Study shows mixing with unvaccinated people poses risk of contracting SARS-CoV-2 infection in vaccinated persons* by Kirti Pandey, *TimesNowNews India (April 25, 2022)*[155]

- *The unvaccinated increase the risk of COVID-19 for the vaccinated when they mingle, Science Media Exchange – Scimex Breaking science news for Australia & New Zealand (April 25, 2022)*[156]

- ***Unvaxxed pose risk of infection for those with shots, research shows as wastewaster suggests COVID soars in Hamilton,*** by Joanna Frketich, *The Hamilton Spectator, (April 26, 2022)[157]*

- ***My Choice? Unvaccinated Pose Outsize Risk to Vaccinated,*** by Kate Johnson, *Medscape Medical News (May 10, 2022)[158]*

The prevailing takeaways from the CMAJ study and spin-off media publications are that unvaccinated people threaten the safety of the vaccinated, they are "drivers" of disease (as interpreted by Dr. William Schaffner, a professor in the Division of Infectious Diseases at the Vanderbilt University School of Medicine in Tennessee, quoted in the Healthline article), and that it's best to "stick to your own kind" (as directly stated in the article by Morgan Lowrie).

In the Global News article by Irelyne Lavery, Fisman explained that models are "simplified versions of reality" and reiterated his findings that the risk goes up in vaccinated people if they mix with unvaccinated people:

> *"We use models in a lot of different ways," said Fisman. "They're just simplified versions of reality."*

> *"When you have a lot of mixing between vaccinated and unvaccinated people, the risk for unvaccinated people actually goes down," said Fisman. "Vaccinated people become a buffer when you have a lot of mixing and risk in vaccinated people goes up."*

The false threat asserted by Fisman, Tuite and Amoako encourages vaccinated people to disassociate with those who chose to forgo COVID-19 vaccination. But the researchers went even further in their attacks against the unvaccinated who, in the opinion of the study's main author, didn't "deserve" to live freely.

The researchers made several inflammatory comparisons and baseless accusations within their CMAJ publication that demean and vilify the unvaccinated. For example, a comparison is made between choosing not to vaccinate and reckless behavior such as driving under the influence of alcohol or other intoxicants. The paper also attributes undue blame to the unvaccinated for poor policy decisions made by our public health care system that led to the cancellation of elective surgeries for cancer and cardiac disease, and that created excessive backlogs. The following excerpt is taken directly from the CMAJ publication:

> ...*acceptance of vaccination is a means of ensuring that greater health care capacity is available for those with other illnesses. For example, in Ontario, capacity for COVID-19 cases in intensive care units was created by cancelling elective surgeries for cancer and cardiac disease, which resulted in extensive backlogs. By contributing to these backlogs, unvaccinated people are creating a risk that those around them may not be able to obtain the care they need and, consequently, the risk they create cannot be considered self-regarding.*

The derisive attitude of the main author, David Fisman, towards those who choose not to get the injections was not born out of any objective scientific analysis. Indeed, his contempt against this group was evident in the early months of the vaccine rollout, as demonstrated in many of his public tweets, including this one back in the summer of 2021 (nine months before the study was published):[159]

"Time for the anti-vaxxers to stay home. The rest of us deserve to get our lives back."

This despite, the day prior, the Ontario Science Table that he served on acknowledging ethical problems with vaccine certificates, coercion and stigma for vaccine hesitant populations and those unable to be vaccinated for medical reasons.[160]

David Fisman has made a great number of disparaging statements about the unvaccinated on his Twitter feed (with over 126.5K followers by the summer of 2022) as well as in interviews discussing the CMAJ study. In the Salon article, "Merely hanging out with unvaccinated people puts the vaccinated at higher risk: study," David Fisman likens the choice to forgo COVID-19 vaccination to choosing to spread tuberculosis, typhoid or syphilis. The direct quote pulled from the article is as follows:

> *"I think it becomes reasonable to use vaccine mandates and passports as a measure that prevents the benefit of vaccines (in those who choose to be*

vaccinated) from being eroded by the choices of others," Fisman continued. "Striking a balance between the rights of individuals and rights of communities is pretty much bread-and-butter public health, so it's unclear to me why this would be contentious. There is no fundamental right to spread tuberculosis, typhoid or syphilis, for example."

In the above quote, Fisman likens *normally-healthy* unvaccinated people to *carriers* of tuberculosis, typhoid, and syphilis. Dr. Fisman, an infectious disease expert, should know that Canadians are not routinely vaccinated against any of these three diseases. In fact, there is no available vaccine for syphilis — all Canadians are "unvaccinated." By his logic, should we all be assumed transmissive and thus confined to pods?

In the CityNews article, "Mixing with unvaccinated increases COVID-19 risk for vaccinated: Study," David Fisman likens the choice not to take the experimental COVID-19 injections to individuals who drive their car 200 kms an hour for fun. The comparison is made to express how vaccine choice impacts the wider community. In that context, the quote appears as follows:

"You may like to drive your car 200 kilometres an hour and think that's fun, but we don't allow you to do that on a highway partly because you can kill and injure yourself, but also because you're creating risk for those around you," said Fisman.

The above quote also appeared in the article written by Morgan Lowrie that was published by the Canadian Press, Toronto Sun, Vancouver Sun, Calgary Sun, Toronto Star, Montreal Gazette, National Observer, National Post, CTV News, Times Colonist, OHS Canada, The Chronicle Journal, CP24, Canoe.com, Castanet.net and elsewhere.

The impact of the study has been far-reaching, cited by countless researchers, medical professionals, columnists, social media podcasters, laypersons and politicians.

Box 3: Related Development

In December 2022, a prominent vaccinologist and viral immunologist filed a lawsuit against David Fisman for tortuous conduct and defamation. In paragraph 200 in the Plaintiff's statement of claim with the Ontario Superior Court of Justice, Fisman along with two other Defendants are accused of:[161]

> 200 (a) Repeated and serial publications of false, malicious, reckless, and, derogatory material, extreme in degree and beyond all possible bounds of decency and tolerance, damaging the Plaintiff and inciting hatred against him;

> 200 (b) Harassment intended to affect the economic interests and reputation and relationships of the Plaintiff.

The claim alleges that Fisman instigated a plot to destroy the Plaintiff's reputation and work following the airing of an interview in May 2021, in which the Plaintiff voiced concerns about the COVID-19 vaccines (paragraphs 58 and 59). The Plaintiff had expressed concerns over potential harms caused by COVID-19 vaccines and suggested the federal government stop giving the injections to children until more studies can be done. The Plaintiff, labelled an "anti-vaxxer" by Fisman, was a career virologist working on the development of a Canadian COVID-19 vaccine at the time.

"Looking very forward to vaccine passports in Canada. Concerns about freedoms? Ok. I think we have a right as a country to be free of disease, death and economic devastation. I think we should be using every carrot and stick legally available to get populations to max vax."

— David Fisman, 10 months before his study[162]

Defrauding Canadians

While the government-funded Fisman study failed to be a serious work of scientific research, it was fit for political purpose: It contrived results to prop up vaccine mandates and restrictions. It provided rationale for governments to undermine an individual's right to bodily autonomy. It vilified those who refused to surrender a Charter right. These elements were by no means subtle. While the vilification of the unvaccinated dominated most headlines, numerous articles highlighted the study's support of vaccine passports, mandates and travel restrictions. Moreover, Fisman openly admitted that his study undermined vaccine choice as an individual right.

The following excerpt is from the previously mentioned spin-off article by Michael Ranger, published in CityNews Everywhere:

> *Researchers say results undermine anti-vaccine arguments, supports vaccine passports*

> *The researchers say this increased risk undermines the message that vaccine choice is best left to the individual, and instead supports enhancing vaccine uptake and limiting access to public spaces for the unvaccinated.*

> *The authors suggest the results of the study stand in stark contrast with the anti-vaccine sentiment that not getting the shot is aligned with the rights of the individual.*

In an interview with Forbes published the same day as the CMAJ article, April 25th 2022, Fisman is quoted as saying that his study's findings support vaccine mandates and passports, and, once again, he compared the unvaccinated to those with tuberculosis and those who drive while intoxicated:

> *Fisman said policies like vaccine mandates or vaccine passports that restrict access to non-essential services such as restaurant dining or public transport seem "reasonable." Such policies are also in line with other regulations designed to protect public health, he said, pointing to compulsory treatment for tuberculosis and restrictions on driving while intoxicated.*

Though the authors advocated for strong, punitive public policy, their study did not involve any of the analysis necessary to draw such an inference. Not only do such policy statements not follow from their analysis, they are well beyond the scope of any simple simulation study. Any suggestion that a hypothetical, provably false simulation can provide any guidance to inform policy, let alone provide strong support for punitive measures, is beyond absurd. Yet, the paper's findings and policy advice were embraced and legitimized by like-minded government officials and institutions such as the University of Toronto. Moreover, CIHR has refused to set the public record straight.

In the aforementioned Forbes article, David Fisman also made specific reference to vaccine mandates for flights and trains when discussing the study findings. The following "critical quote" was highlighted in the Forbes article:

> *"Vaccinated individuals have a right not to have their efforts to protect themselves undermined," Fisman said, stressing that the findings are "very supportive" of vaccine mandates for flights and trains.*

Throughout the pandemic, Canadians had been expected to forfeit their own moral compasses and logic centers and to instead "follow the science" as dictated by mainstream experts. They were expected to do so again.

The study was published in a peer-reviewed medical journal by credentialed epidemiologists, complete with the full suite of messaging that the Liberals required for their discriminatory measures. All that was needed was sufficient mainstream media coverage and official recognition by Parliament. Media was more than happy to oblige and the story was taken up by at least 90 online outlets with dissemination to the public beginning within hours of the CMAJ publication. Then a few days later, with the study in hand, the Parliamentary Secretary to the Minister of Health was ready to defend the travel restrictions when called on to do so in the House of Commons. The April 29th exchange went as follows:[163]

> *Mr. Blaine Calkins (Red Deer—Lacombe, CPC): "Madam Speaker, if the NDP-Liberals will not follow the province's lead and give unvaccinated Canadians their rights back, maybe they will follow our international partners... Switzerland and Greece are removing all travel-related restrictions*

next week and virtually no other country requires them for domestic travel for their citizens, so why will the government not follow the science?"

Mr. Adam van Koeverden (Parliamentary Secretary to the Minister of Health and to the Minister of Sport, Lib.): "Madam Speaker, I thank my hon. colleague for giving me the opportunity to highlight a recent study indicating that unfortunately the unvaccinated continue to disproportionately risk the safety of those vaccinated against COVID-19."

While Mr. van Koeverden was eager to showcase the faux Fisman study hot off the press, the months and months of real-world data published on the official Government of Ontario website failed to draw his attention. The real data indicated that the early-year Omicron surge was dominated by infections amongst the fully vaccinated, not the unvaccinated (as was shown in Figures 5 and 7). Moreover, by the spring of 2022 it was the boosted who had disproportionately more infections than others (as shown in Figure 11).

Figure 11: COVID-19 Incident Rates by Vaccination Status
Ontario Data: March 17, 2022 to June 10, 2022

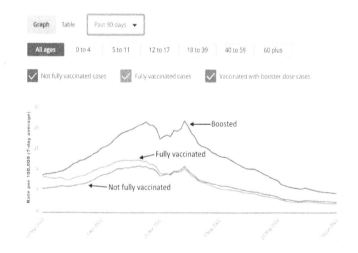

Box 4: Ban the Boosted?

Publicly available data from the official Government of Ontario COVID-19 website showed that incident rates amongst persons who received their COVID-19 booster shot far exceeded those of the not fully vaccinated and double vaccinated individuals in 2022, up until the government stopped tracking cases by vaccination status. This trend was also observed in other countries.

In the UK, reported infection rates amongst individuals vaccinated with at least three doses far exceeded unvaccinated infection rates for all adult age groups throughout the early months of 2022.[164] This trend of negative effectiveness worsened month over month until the data stopped being reported at the end of March, at which time the incident rates amongst the boosted were 3 to 5 times those of the unvaccinated for most adult age groups. The UKHSA provided several reasons why the layperson shouldn't calculate raw vaccine effectiveness rates based on their official data. Indeed, it takes a great amount of statistical sorcery to go from an effectiveness rate hovering around -400% into positive territory and not everyone is gifted with that kind of magic. Best to leave it to the "experts."

Brutal results in the USA study by Shrestha et al. (2023) indicate that the higher the number of vaccines previously received, the higher the risk of contracting COVID-19. The finding is certainly cause for concern and warrants further investigation.[165]

The Search for Positive Efficacy

Transmission studies read more and more like statistical fishing expeditions with researchers desperately seeking out the fleeting conditions (and manipulations) under which the vaccines can be shown to demonstrate a modicum of positive efficacy. It reeks of desperation, so much so that one is left to wonder just how much of the original claim of 95% efficacy was a mere statistical illusion.[166] Either way, such fleeting benefit, perceived or real, is of little use if it leads to greater transmission down the road.

"I cannot imagine that we're going to let a small and unreasonable minority hold back our economy and trash our healthcare system this fall. Vaccine passports now."

— David Fisman, 9 months before his study[167]

Objectivity is crucial in scientific research. However, the researchers' overt bias and contempt towards the unvaccinated permeated every facet of their study. Moreover, statements in the CMAJ paper and comments made by Fisman in follow-up interviews demonstrate that the study was motivated by political ideology.

> *Fisman said the idea for study came a few months ago amid the debate around vaccine passports and vaccine mandates.*
>
> *"We thought what was missing from that conversation was, what are the rights of vaccinated people to be protected from unvaccinated people?" he said.*
>
> *...Fisman said the results, from a purely "utilitarian" perspective, provide justification for the implementation of public health measures such as vaccine passports and vaccine mandates.*
>
> *— Taken from the article by Morgan Lowrie, Canadian Press, April 25, 2022*

Despite having acknowledged receipt of criticisms from dozens of researchers and scientists regarding the incorrect interpretation of the study's results and concerns that the research was stoking hatred, Fisman, Amoako and Tuite have thus far failed to correct the record.

My own efforts to have the fraudulent paper retracted and the record set straight regarding the fictitious findings are documented in the accompanying supplementary guide. I pushed through the formal complaint process for each of the three institutes involved. In all instances,

I provided a detailed account of the problematic statements in the research publication. The official complaint process of these institutions specify that they apprise the study's researchers of *all* correspondence, yet the researchers have failed to take any action, have not retracted their paper nor the faux findings.

As demonstrated throughout this book, the fraudulent study by David Fisman, Afia Amoako and Ashleigh Tuite, has generated a massive trail of misinformation, resulting in the propagation of fear, mistrust, and derisive attitudes towards an unfairly targeted segment of the population. Moreover, the authors have leveraged the false statements in an attempt to defraud millions of Canadians of basic rights and freedoms.

The actions and statements made by the authors have resulted in sustained anguish and have contributed to incremental financial losses for the travel industry, employees impacted by the federal vaccine mandate, and individuals unable to return to work in other sectors because their employers falsely believed (and many still believe) that the unvaccinated pose a greater risk to their workforce. The harm has been massive.

The harms from the fraudulent study and actions of Fisman and his two colleagues were not limited to those who had chosen to forgo COVID-19 vaccination. Individuals may have been swayed to get vaccinated or accept additional doses, the cumulative effects of which were, and still are, largely unknown.

> *So gratified to hear from a colleague that our @cmaj paper led to one of their relatives changing their mind about vaccination.*
>
> — *David Fisman, April 29, 2022 (Twitter)*

Over-selling people on a drug that comes with serious risks while ignoring potential harms is dangerous. This is especially true for individuals who have little to benefit from the drug and are at increased risk of long-term harms, such as the young.

Children and healthy young adults have little to nothing to gain from the vaccines and are more likely to bear the risk of any long-term adverse health consequences that may come to fruition. It is unethical and reckless to use coercive and deceitful methods to increase COVID-19 vaccine uptake amongst this group.[168] Moreover, the disease risk for the majority of working-aged individuals was known from the onset to be fairly low and manageable. Fisman and his colleagues have claimed that their study took a "utilitarian" approach. However, misrepresenting the effectiveness of a new drug is not done for the "greater good" and a utilitarian approach isn't one that sacrifices the health and safety of the young or the workforce.

By September 2022, several European countries had stopped offering or recommending mRNA vaccines to healthy young children, including the UK, Sweden, Finland and Norway.[169] Denmark had halted COVID-19 vaccinations for low-risk people under age 50.[170]

David Fisman, however, continued to promote general vaccine mandates and vaccine uptake amongst children and healthy young adults.

> *...vaccine mandates continue to be an important tool to promote health equity, and protect the right of vaccinated individuals not to have their efforts to protect their health undermined*
>
> — *David Fisman, Aug 24, 2022 (Twitter)*

> *Please get your kids vaccinated. Make sure they're up to date with as many vaccine doses as they're eligible for.*
>
> — *David Fisman, Sept 2, 2022 (Twitter)*

Scientific fraud is not a victimless undertaking. But even in the face of extreme research misconduct — complete data fabrication — journals and institutions often fail to acknowledge the fraud committed against them and the wider community. In a 2015 article published in the CMAJ entitled "Scientific misconduct or criminal offence?" Dr. Zulfiqar Bhutta, co-director of research for the Centre for Global Child Health at The Hospital for Sick Children in Toronto, expressed the view that the research community does an inadequate job of policing itself.[171] He, and others in the scientific community, were of the mindset that, given the huge ramifications of research fraud on public health and clinical practice, researchers who commit fraud should face criminal charges in court.

> *If someone defrauds tax payers with research money and falsifies data or falsifies entire research results, it is no different than any other form of similar economic crime.*
>
> — *Dr. Bhutta, Co-director of research, SickKids (CMAJ, 2015)*

In a 2014 BMJ article, Bhutta also cited the damage to global vaccination coverage that has been caused by fraudulent research.[172] Testimony by Dr. Kevin Bardosh before a US Government Subcommittee on COVID-19 discussed how vaccine mandates and passports have destroyed many people's trust in public health institutions, which has increased vaccine hesitancy. He has no doubt that, because of these measures, there will be increased distrust and resistance next time there's a pandemic.[173] The study by Fisman, Tuite and Amoako has created a situation whereby provably fraudulent research was used to justify vaccine mandates and restrictions, scapegoat those who did not comply, and coerce greater vaccine uptake. Just how much has that double or triple whammy impacted vaccine hesitancy?

Under the laws in the Criminal Code of Canada Section 380, it is illegal and unlawful for a person to use fraudulent means, whether or not it is a false pretense, to defraud the public or any person, whether ascertained or not, of any property, money or valuable security or any service.

As mentioned in Chapter 4, differentiating between intentional fraud and general incompetence can be challenging. Indeed, some have argued that the time and resources required to meet the high burden of proof for a criminal conviction is an inefficient way to improve science and that stewardship is best left with research institutions. That very sentiment was voiced by CIHR's former executive director of the Secretariat on Responsible Conduct of Research in the 2015 CMAJ article regarding misconduct.

The convictions of research integrity by CIHR, CMAJ and U of T were put to the test with Fisman's fraud. How they responded to the allegations is covered in Chapter 9. The OPP's response to the evidence is discussed in Chapter 10.

A Tool for Coercion & Extortion

Under Section 346 of the Criminal Code, extortion — the practice of obtaining something through coercion without reasonable justification or excuse — is a crime.

Lacking any other scientific evidence that vaccine mandates and passports would effectively reduce community transmission, Fisman's fraudulent study was offered up as the sole justification to extend federal travel restrictions.

With the implementation of vaccine passports and mandates, Canadians were given an ultimatum: get injected with a series of experimental genetic COVID-19 vaccines or face exclusion from public venues such as gyms, restaurants and theatres; exclusion from sport teams and social gatherings; possible job loss or termination of income; denied access to post-secondary education; and, be banned from travel by air, train or boat. The demand for vaccination and consequences of non-compliance were done in the name of "science" despite a notable lack of any such science being presented.

In the fall of 2021, the Trudeau government enacted a policy banning unvaccinated travellers over the age of 12 from boarding a plane or passenger train in Canada. However, when called to testify in legal proceedings, public officials responsible for the restrictive travel policies admitted to a lack of scientific justification for the measures imposed. The cross-examination of top government officials during a Charter challenge revealed that the Public Health Agency of Canada (PHAC) did not include vaccine requirements in its COVID-19 mitigation strategy for air travellers because the scientific evidence did not support that it would be effective. Indeed, neither PHAC nor Health Canada had recommended vaccine mandates for air travel.[174]

As testified by PHAC epidemiologist Dr. Lisa Waddell, data indicated there wasn't much risk of transmission on airplanes.[175] She had written a study for PHAC stating as much. During further cross examinations it was revealed that Transport Canada had made the conscious decision not to grant exemptions for travel on compassionate grounds in order to "incentivize" Canadians to get vaccinated.[176] Then, during the Public Order Emergency Commission (POEC) hearings, Deputy Prime Minister Chrystia Freeland admitted that the true purpose of the cross-border regulations on truckers was to compel as many Canadians as possible to get vaccinated.[177] These testimonials from top government officials indicate that the true goal of the mandates and restrictions was not for public safety via reduced transmission, but was to coerce all Canadians to take a vaccine that millions clearly did not want or need. Without scientific justification, these acts of coercion are akin to extortion.

David Fisman and his two colleagues produced fraudulent research under the guise of science that was used by politicians to justify their highly restrictive measures.

In addition to advocating for coercive public policy and providing possible cover for decisions made by government officials, the researchers conducted coercive tactics of their own. More specifically, the researchers engaged in menaces and made unfounded accusations aimed to coerce and/ or intimidate people into accepting new, additional or ongoing vaccination in order to avoid damage to reputation and public shaming. The ultimate goal, to increase vaccine uptake, is an activity which the main researcher, David Fisman, has personal stakes (as discussed in Chapter 3).

CHAPTER 8

The Outcry: Rebukes by the Scientific Community

"The combination of deeply flawed modelling, moral condemnation and politicisation should be sufficient to retract a paper published in Canada's preeminent medical journal. Unfortunately, the damage has already been done."
— *J. Doidge, A. de Figueiredo, T. Lemmens, K. Bardosh*

Rebukes of the Fisman et al. study came fast and furious with more than a dozen eLetters to the editor posted on the CMAJ website by almost two dozen researchers within the first week of the paper's release. How many eLetters CMAJ received in total remains unclear. The journal is not obliged to post them all. For example, the letter I submitted in the early days of May 2022 never appeared on the journal's designated response webpage.

Below are quotes taken from a sample of the eLetters posted to CMAJ's website for public viewing.

Excerpt 1: taken from the Letter to the CMAJ editor submitted by York N. Hsiang [MB ChB, MHSc., FRCSC], Vascular surgeon, University of British Columbia (Posted on: 27 April 2022).

> *As there is abundant real-world data, why they would choose a mathematical model is unclear… Promotion of poor research such as this leads to further*

stigmatization and division in society. We challenge the CMAJ to retract this study or issue a correction in their next publication.

Excerpt 2: taken from the Letter to the CMAJ editor submitted by Pooya Kazemi [MD, MSc], Anesthesiologist, Island Health (Posted on: 29 April 2022).

Given the serious flaws of this modelling study, it is unfortunate that it has received wide media attention. The media narratives being sold based on this study are troubling, because they do not reflect reality but are causing further societal division in Canada.

Excerpt 3: taken from the Letter to the CMAJ editor submitted by: James Doidge, PhD, Medical statistician; Alex de Figueiredo, Statistician; Trudo Lemmens, Professor and Scholl Chair in Health Law and Policy; Kevin Bardosh, Applied medical anthropologist (Posted on: 28 April 2022).

The findings are predetermined by the authors' own model design choices; something that should never occur in science. That the authors make strong ethical and political claims that feed existing social polarization makes the flawed design even more problematic...

It is especially problematic that a modelling paper so detached from reality contains such explicit and strong condemnation of 'the unvaccinated'.

Excerpt 4: taken from the Letter to the CMAJ editor submitted by Mary Lynch, MD, FRCPC (Posted on: 1 May 2022).

There are significant problems with this study.

Starting with the title: The title implies that there was actual mixing of populations in the study, this was not the case... Real world experience using the most recent Ontario statistics demonstrates that it is the vaccinated who are at most risk of having or being hospitalized with COVID....

This article has received widespread media attention and is spreading inaccurate information with potential to further polarize Canadians and others. Consideration should be given to retraction with an apology.

Excerpt 5: taken from the Letter to the CMAJ editor submitted by Edward J Bosveld [B.A., M.B.A.], Professor, Public Policy, Redeemer University (Posted on: 2 May 2022).

> *Inflated estimates of vaccine effectiveness, complete disregard of waning immunity, and underestimation of natural immunity among the unvaccinated are all used to support the claim that the minority is dangerous to the majority and that "mixing" with such disease-carriers is risky. While there is considerable historical precedent for such scapegoating, the CMAJ should reconsider whether it is prudent and ethical to publish models which support this type of discrimination.*

Excerpt 6: taken from the Letter to the CMAJ editor submitted by Jennifer M. Grant, Infectious Diseases Specialist, Clinical Associate Professor, University of British Columbia; Matt S Strauss, Medical officer of health, Acting medical officer of health, Haldimand-Norfolk; Martha Fulford, Infectious Diseases specialist, McMaster University; Roy Eappen, Endocrinologist, McGill University (Posted on: 30 April 2022).

> *Using numbers that are more realistic in the study model reverses the paper's conclusions and better match the observed data.*

According to CMAJ, letters to the editor represent the post-publication peer review of an article. In this case, the letters were scathing, unanimously depicting the study as seriously flawed with invalid conclusions — in fact opposite reality, as pointed out by many. Concerns about the study sowing societal division and stigmatizing/scapegoating a portion of the population were expressed by many researchers and medical doctors; several letters requested the study be retracted. But did the journal issue a retraction or undertake any corrective measure? — *No.*

The criticisms of the flawed study didn't end there. Many researchers, medical practitioners and concerned citizens took to social media denouncing the study and calling out the bogus findings. While alternative media outlets and some local radio shows took notice of the backlash, the major mainstream outlets that had sensationalized the study's faux findings failed to acknowledge the problems and they did not issue corrections.

> *This paper, it is very divisive and it spreads a lot of disinformation that's verifiable.*
>
> — *Eric Payne, MD pediatric neurologist and clinical researcher [Western Standard Podcast, 1 min mark]*[178]

The range of expertise of those critiquing the Fisman et al. paper is telling: scientists and physicians across numerous specialties, current and retired, from infectious diseases specialists and clinical researchers to neurologist to vascular surgeon, endocrinologist, computational expert, viral immunologist, physicists, statisticians, professionals in health law and public policy... the list goes on. This "scientific" model fails across the board.

Table 1 provides a summary of the eLetters that were posted on the CMAJ website in response to Fisman, Tuite, and Amoako's fraudulent study within just one week of the paper's publication. Table 2 provides a sample of critiques by other researchers and physicians that have been shared online. Also included are comments from a lawyer made during a podcast discussing how the fraudulent paper is meant to influence the mind of the judiciary and targeted court cases.

The quotes in this section along with the materials presented in Tables 1 and 2 make clear that the work by Fisman, Tuite and Amoako fails the slightest scrutiny. Indeed, the study is likely to be considered junk science by any competent researcher who takes the time to delve into the publication.

But such effort isn't made by most people. Indeed, the masses are informed by media and most individuals trust that peer-reviewed medical journals, such as CMAJ, publish credible research. Unfortunately, the low-quality and fraudulent nature of the study didn't seem to matter to the journal, the media, nor politicians looking for any morsel to "validate" the discriminatory vaccine policies and restrictions. The paper had served its purpose.

As barrister & solicitor Jeffrey Rath explained during an online podcast (Table 2), from his perspective the Fisman study was a propaganda piece intended to influence the court case for travel restrictions against the unvaccinated and to propagate false narratives in the public square — to pretend what they were doing made sense despite real science and data indicating the diametric opposite.

Unless researchers are held accountable for their research and the harm created by false statements and reckless recommendations, this plunge into the world of contrived mathematical fantasy is likely to continue.

The last entry in Table 2, a podcast featuring Dr. Ralph Behrens' letter, hits on a very troubling trend. Namely, the increased reliance on mathematical modelling to inform policy. Dr. Behrens' comments reinforce many of the concerns regarding the degradation of scientific evidence discussed in Chapter 5. From the podcast:

> *We have yet to observe any real accuracy nor public health benefit to the multiple computer modelled declarations or the policies they generate to date…*
>
> *Since the beginning of the SARS-CoV-2 pandemic, the level of academic rigour, integrity, and quality used to support mandates, restrictions, and public health guidance has drastically diminished.*
>
> *We are forced to adhere to observational data and models, which would fail scrutiny in any first-year medical epidemiology course as the gold standards for determining efficacy and effectiveness. Appallingly, this same evidence is being used to guide and dictate policies, which have caused irreversible damage to adolescents, families, careers, and our health care system.*
>
> — *Ralph Behrens, MD*

Table 1: Summary of eLetters posted on the CMAJ website in response to the Fisman et al. study (week of April 25, 2022 – May 2, 2022).[179]

Researcher	Main Criticisms of Fisman et al Study
*Jennifer M. Grant, Infectious Diseases Specialist, Clinical Associate Professor, University of British Columbia	Invalid/incorrect results opposite real-world; Unjustified policy directives; Invalid input parameters & assumptions.
Matt S Strauss, Medical officer of health, Acting medical officer of health, Haldimand-Norfolk	
Martha Fulford, Infectious Diseases specialist, McMaster University	
Roy Eappen, Endocrinologist, McGill University	
*James C Doidge [PhD], Medical statistician, Intensive Care National Audit and Research Centre; and London School of Hygiene and Tropical Medicine	Deeply flawed modelling, detached from reality; Findings are predetermined by the authors; Fosters social division, misplaced anger and blame; Inappropriate and inadequate comments regarding health care resources; Request retraction.
Alex de Figueiredo, Statistician	
Trudo Lemmens, Professor and Scholl Chair in Health Law and Policy	
Kevin Bardosh, Applied medical anthropologist	
Edward J Bosveld [B.A., M.B.A.], Professor, Public Policy, Redeemer University	Flawed inputs used to vilify a minority.

*Denis G. Rancourt [BSc, MSc, PhD (Physics)], Researcher, Ontario Civil Liberties Association (ocla.ca)	Main conclusion does not follow from their model;
Joseph Hickey, Executive Director	Flawed model and interpretation.
Jesse Aumond-Beaupre [BASc], Engineer, Université du Québec en Abitibi-Témiscamingue	Conclusions do not match public data from UK, Scotland, Sweden, Denmark, Ontario, Quebec, Iceland, etc. Erroneous input parameters.
Stephenson B Strobel [MD MA Msc], PhD Candidate; Emergency Physician, Brooks School of Public Policy, Cornell University; Niagara Health	Model doesn't represent the real world; Invalid, coercive policy conclusions that may violate individual freedoms.
Dena L. Schanzer [M.Sc., P.Stat.], Statistician, infectious diseases, Public Health Agency of Canada (retired)	Main finding of the study is opposite real-world trends.
York N. Hsiang [MB ChB, MHSc., FRCSC], Vascular surgeon, University of British Columbia	Poor (unscientific) research; Stigmatizes and divides society; Request retraction of study.
Pooya Kazemi [MD, MSc], Anesthesiologist, Island Health	Serious flaws in study; The media narratives do not reflect reality and are causing further societal division in Canada.
Steve Blitzer [MD], Physician, Medical Centre / Mackenzie Health	Flawed mathematical model.

Edward E. Rylander [MD], Physician, IHI Family Medicine Residency	Invalid/Poor input assumption.
Ovidiu Lungu [PhD], scientist	Title of the paper and the presentation of the findings in mass-media is misleading; Results are misinterpreted as being based on data collected from real people.
Mary Lynch [MD FRCPC], Pain Medicine, Dalhousie University	The title implies that there was actual mixing of populations in the study; Conclusions not consistent (opposite) with real world experience; Inaccurate assumptions; Significant conflict of interest with the lead author; Pejorative, inaccurate description 'unvaccinated'; Widespread polarizing misinformation; Request retraction with an apology.
Richard Schabas [MD MHSc FRCPC], public health physician (retired)	Flawed model assumptions, invalid conclusions.
Paul Carr [MD], Emergency physician, Lakeridge Health	Overstated vaccine efficacy (model assumption).

Table 2: Sample of Online Critiques of the Fisman, Tuite, and Amoako fraudulent study

Researcher & Article Title	Main Criticisms of Fisman et al Study
Byram Bridle, PhD Associate Professor of Viral Immunology in the Department of Pathobiology at the University of Guelph: "Fiction Disguised as Science to Promote Hatred: Disinformation Must Be Called Out."[180]	Critically flawed study & model: numerous issues; Promotes hatred, segregation, and the potential development of harmful policies; Call for paper to be retracted.
Jessica Rose, BSc. Applied Mathematics, MSc. Immunology, PhD Computational Biology: Call for retraction of paper entitled: "Impact of population mixing between vaccinated and unvaccinated subpopulations on infectious disease dynamics: implications for SARS-CoV-2 transmission."	There is no scientific merit to the study; Creates division in society; Poor/unreliable model; Model parameters not based on real data and opposite to what real data indicates; Who were the reviewers? This paper should not have been published.
Eric Payne, MD pediatric neurologist and clinical researcher: [Video] "Calgary medical specialist and lawyer refute misinformation on unvaxxed being COVID spreaders"	Divisive, spreads disinformation; Faulty, biased, nonsense model; Study conclusions opposite to real-world observations.

Jeffrey Rath, B.A. (Hons.), LL.B. (Hons.) BARRISTER & SOLICITOR, Taking Back Our Freedoms Board Director: [Video] As above with Eric Payne.	Propaganda piece intended to impact mind of judiciary and court cases; The study was meant to impact the court case for travel restrictions against the unvaccinated; The study infers outside authors area of expertise; Meant to propagate false narratives in public square to pretend what they are doing makes sense when real science and data says diametric opposite.
Ralph Behrens, MD in British Columbia: Podcast: "Your Voice: Study on risk of mixing with unvaccinated based on 'unproven and subjective' models"	Unproven and subjective model; Conclusions incorrect and biased; A deceptive study, used to intentionally mislead the public, fraught with glaring omissions and misassumptions not reflective of current data; Fisman has multiple and significant conflicts of interest; Promotes further stigmatization and division in our society. Call for a retraction of the study.

Response: CMAJ Embraces Pseudoscience

Pseudoscience consists of statements, beliefs, or practices that claim to be both scientific and factual, but are incompatible with the scientific method. (Oxford English Dictionary, second edition 1989)

Given the many obvious issues with Fisman's pseudoscientific study, as well as the timing of its release and the rapidity at which it was taken up by mass media, it is clear more was driving the effort than grand incompetency. The big question is: who knowingly facilitated the creation or dissemination of the fraudulent material?

> As a researcher who has published and reviewed many scientific papers, I can tell you the article by (David) Fisman et al. is the worst one that I have ever seen.

> —Byram Bridle, PhD Viral Immunology[181]

The first step towards answering the big question is uncovering how such a flawed study could have passed a legitimate peer review process and have been published by a Canadian medical journal. Reputable journals generally screen for obvious scientific flaws and potential breaches of ethics to safeguard research integrity and human rights.

So, what happened?

In an effort to gauge CMAJ's input, the next chapter compares the original preprint submitted to the journal to versions of the paper as it moved through the review process towards publication.

One of the biggest problems with the published version of the paper was that it was widely misinterpreted as being based on data collected from *real people* as opposed to a contrived, self-fulfilling simulation exercise. As shown in the next chapter, targeted changes made during the revision process indicate there was a deliberate attempt to foster this misinterpretation.

Over the course of the CMAJ peer-reviewed process, a critically flawed, heavily biased mathematical modelling study became an overtly fraudulent and defamatory work of hate science.

CMAJ is hopelessly incriminated in the deception. That in itself is scandalous. That the University of Toronto refused to investigate the researchers for fabricating "facts" based on contrived models while selecting David Fisman to take a lead role in modelling future pandemics is equally unsettling. Fisman has demonstrated significant influence in shaping Canada's COVID-19 pandemic response. With his infamous study funded by the federal government and exploited by top Liberal politicians, the possibility of political involvement in the deception cannot be ruled out.

In addition to the preprint version comparisons, the next chapter examines the responses by CMAJ, the University of Toronto and CIHR to repeated requests for investigation into the Fisman et al. study and what those responses imply.

CHAPTER 9

The Gatekeepers

"In every facet of life, there are gatekeepers. Learn to get around them."

— Jillian Michaels, American fitness expert & businesswoman (1974–)

The Fisman et al. paper possesses all the characteristics of pseudoscience. Yet, it supposedly passed the peer review process by a top Canadian medical journal, was rubber-stamped by Canada's preeminent university and was fully backed by CIHR, Canada's federal funding agency for health research.

Box 5: Pseudoscience
Non-Science Posing as Science

Characteristics of pseudoscience: contradictory and exaggerated claims; reliance on confirmation bias; absence of systematic practices when developing hypotheses; lack of openness to evaluation by other experts; and, continued adherence long after the pseudo-scientific hypotheses have been discredited.

Pseudoscience is often shown to be "fact-resistant."

If the many red flags had somehow been missed by all three institutions prior to publication, they were certainly brought to their attention in the weeks that followed, by myself and at least dozens of other researchers. Indeed, I provided a rather detailed 20 page critique to all three organizations that demonstrated the complete lack of scientific quality and integrity of the Fisman study. However, the triplet of researchers and all three organizations have shown an unwillingness to accept strongly supported factual statements — a telltale hallmark of pseudoscience.

This Chapter provides an overview of the responses from each of the three organizations to the critiques I provided them, and the responses to my requests to have the publication retracted or, at the very least, corrected. My full critique of the study along with all letters and correspondences with the institutions are provided in the supplementary reference, *Fisman's Fraud: The Accomplices*.

The Problematic CMAJ Review Process

Q: Did the Fisman et al. paper actually pass a legitimate peer-review process?

Many scientists have openly questioned how the Fisman et al. paper — a incredibly flawed piece of hate science — could have passed a true scientific review process and gone on to be published by a Canadian medical journal.

> *You could get kicked out of university for this and would most certainly fail your modeling course.*
>
> —*Jessica Rose, BSc. Applied Math, MSc. Immunology, PhD Computational Biology*[182]

Apart from an automated response and a form letter acknowledging my initial eLetter submission and a follow-up email, CMAJ did not engage in any meaningful correspondence. Their non-response prompted me to scrutinize the paper's road to publication and CMAJ's involvement in the disinformation.

Though CMAJ has an anonymous peer review process, a quick online search turns up three versions of the paper:

- A December 16th, 2021 preprint: The earliest online version of the paper prior to peer review.[183]

- A March 4th, 2022 revised preprint: The second version, revised after peer review by CMAJ.[184]

- The April 25th, 2022 final publication: The final (accepted) peer-reviewed version widely cited by national and international media outlets.[185]

By comparing the original document submitted to the journal to later versions, insight into what transpired during the CMAJ review process can be gained. Shockingly, with each iteration the number of problematic statements increased. While the same fundamentally flawed model underpinned the analysis of all three papers, the level of bias, misrepresentation and political pandering grew as the paper moved through peer review.

The first preprint was completed just as COVID-19 cases were ramping up in Canada, prior to the Omicron surge. When the surge hit and cases spiked to new heights, concerns mounted regarding the apparent reduction in vaccine effectiveness. The revised preprint posted in March and the final paper published in April shifted focus to address the Omicron variant, quell vaccine doubt, and encourage COVID-19 vaccine uptake. Key revisions made during the peer-review process included:

1. Countering the Omicron surge with reassuring claims and biased estimates;

2. Disguising the fake simulation as a real-world occurrence;

3. Adding derogatory comparisons against the unvaccinated;

4. Using stronger, more definitive language that pits vaccinated against unvaccinated.

Together, these revisions aimed to transform a hypothetical demonstration of how vaccination choice affects the community as a whole to a rewrite of history masking vaccine failure, scapegoating the unvaccinated and pushing for government overreach.

AIM OF THE ORIGINAL PREPRINT (Dec. 2021)

The overarching message of the first preprint was that not getting vaccinated negatively impacts infectious disease dynamics and, as such, the choice shouldn't be left to the individual. Indeed, the aim of the simulation exercise was to undermine an individual's right to bodily autonomy by (fictitiously) demonstrating that unvaccinated individuals create a disproportionate risk to the community.

Under the paper's critically flawed modelling and faulty assumptions, the authors threw their support behind draconian action — when it comes to vaccination, the principle of self-governance need not apply and, instead, prohibiting the unvaccinated from socializing and other coercive tactics is the way forward.

Unlike subsequent versions, the original preprint version of the paper more clearly indicated the study was a simple mathematical modelling exercise and was not a real-world study. This first preprint was posted on December 16th, just as the Omicron wave was rising. The simulation described therein was parameterized to the Delta variant though; transmission dynamics under the Omicron variant wasn't modelled at all.

Immediately following the submission of the preprint, the Omicron variant took hold in Ontario and the rest of Canada. COVID-19 cases surged. The authors revised their paper, re-calibrating their model and adjusting their messaging to account for the dominant Omicron variant and counter growing doubts about vaccine effectiveness. Key revisions under CMAJ's guidance are provided in what follows.

Revision Theme #1: Countering the Omicron Surge

In the March preprint and final publication, the Omicron variant took center stage. The authors acknowledged that the increased transmissibility of the Omicron variant may undermine some vaccine gains (such as reducing severity and disrupting transmission), but provided assurances that the vaccines were still highly effective. More specifically:

- The researchers stated that: "provision of booster vaccine doses may restore vaccination to a high level of potency."

- The researchers claimed: "Boosting with mRNA vaccines appears to restore vaccine effectiveness at least temporarily against Omicron, and it is likely that the higher vaccine effectiveness estimates used in our model will be relevant to public policy as booster campaigns are scaled up in Canada and elsewhere."

These assurances were bolstered by the overly optimistic and unrealistic choice of model parameters (as detailed in the supplementary guide). Recall that model parameters for Omicron effectiveness were chosen in a manner that simulated trends *contrary* to what publicly available official government COVID-19 data was showing.

Stripped away from the final publication was any mention that the pandemic appeared to be waning or that unvaccinated individuals could possibly show lower COVID-19 incidence rates at any time. For example, the following statement appeared in the December preprint, but not the later versions:

> *Post-epidemic incidence was lower among unvaccinated individuals than among vaccinated individuals, as the explosive epidemic among unvaccinated individuals resulted in a lower fraction of these individuals in the susceptible compartment as the epidemic waned.*

In the March preprint the following statement acknowledged the pandemic was waning, but was removed in the final version:

> *While our focus here is on a pandemic that now appears to be waning...*

The above statement's appearance in the March preprint confirms the researchers were aware of real-world data trends and that their study focus was on the (recent) past Omicron wave and not some future outbreak. The researchers' choice to not validate their model using real-world observations and instead publish fabricated results that countered the failure of COVID-19 vaccines in curtailing transmission may be construed by some to be an egregious act of medical fraud.

In snuffing out any hint that vaccine benefit may not be as rosy as portrayed by their study, the researchers nullified the only disclaimer they had regarding their model's inadequacy. The following limitation was included in all three versions:

> *The simplicity of our model is both a strength (as it provides a system that is transparent and easily modified to explore the impact of uncertainty) and a weakness, because it does not precisely simulate a real-world pandemic process in all its complexity.*

It's a vague a statement, true of *any* mathematical model, so in that sense it's quite empty and benign. However, while the December preprint provided no indication of how the model limitations might impact results, the following misdirected claim was added to subsequent versions:

> *For instance, we modelled vaccine effectiveness against infection but not the additional benefits of vaccination for preventing severe illness… We have also likely underestimated vaccine benefit in this model, as we have not attempted to capture the impact of vaccines on prevention of forward transmission by vaccinated, infected individuals; this effect appears to be substantial.*

So, the only "weaknesses" to which readers were alerted served to strengthen the study's foregone conclusion that COVID-19 vaccines offer tremendous benefit – no risks, no uncertainty, no inconvenient real-world observations to spoil the fantasy. The level of bias was extreme, to the point of incredulous.

As another example of the researchers' ability to turn weaknesses into raving benefits is their claim that when vaccines confer imperfect immunity (as we've seen with the Omicron variant), non-vaccination heightens risk for vaccinated populations. That is, the more imperfect the vaccine the more we should vaccinate!

Revision Theme #2: Disguising the Fake as Real

A key problem with the study is that its results, which are contrary to what was actually observed in Ontario, have been widely misinterpreted as being based on data collected from real people. Indeed, the study has been used to overwrite reality, pit vaccinated people against unvaccinated people, and to lobby support for vaccine uptake at the expense of constitutional rights and freedoms. Targeted changes made during the revision process indicate a deliberate attempt to foster this misinterpretation. The revision process obscured the nonfactual nature of the study in three ways:

TACTIC 1: PEOPLE, PEOPLE, PEOPLE

Simulated entities in the oversimplified model were referred to as flesh-and-blood people who chose to put others at increased risk. Despite a complete absence of people or real-world observations in their study, the term "people" was purposefully inserted into the revised preprint and further emphasized in the published version:

- In the December 2021 preprint, the term "people" is used only **once**.

- In the March 2022 revised preprint, "people" is mentioned **five times**.

- In the April 2022 publication, "people" is mentioned **76 TIMES**!

TACTIC 2: GET RID OF ALL THAT MODELLING JARGON

In the first preprint, the nature of the study as a mathematical simulation was more apparent; differential equations and technical verbiage were presented in the main body of the document. In subsequent versions, equations, or any mention thereof, were moved to the technical appendix along with the schematic "stock and flow" diagram of the model. This increased the paper's appeal to non-scientists.

TACTIC 3: VISUALIZING REAL WORLD TRANSMISSION

The fairly technical description of transmission dynamics in the December preprint was, in the two subsequent versions, replaced with a conceptual discussion of how transmission might play out in the real world. Compare the phrasing between the three drafts:

- December preprint: "**The model** was subdivided into two connected sub-populations: vaccinated individuals and unvaccinated individuals (Figure 1 [a "stock and flow" **model schematic**]). **The model** is governed by the following **ordinary differential equations,** where i represents the vaccination status of the group, and j represents vaccination status of contacts..."

  ○ Equations and a somewhat technical description of model parameters and transmission dynamics followed.

- March revised preprint: "**The model** represents individuals as residing in three possible "compartments": susceptible to infection (S), infected and infectious (I), and recovered from infection with immunity (R). The compartments are divided to reflect two connected sub-populations: vaccinated individuals and unvaccinated individuals."

  ○ A less technical, more conceptual description of transmission followed with "effective contact" visualized as "sharing air" with an infective case.

- April publication: "**People** are represented as residing in 3 possible "compartments:" susceptible to infection (S), infected and infectious (I), and recovered from infection with immunity (R). We divided the compartments to reflect 2 connected subpopulations: vaccinated and unvaccinated **people.** Susceptible **people**..."

  ○ Transmission dynamics are described similar to the March conceptualization, i.e. sharing air with an infective case for a duration sufficient to permit transmission.

Revision Theme #3: Adding Derogatory Comparisons

While overt bias favoring COVID-19 vaccination was present in all three versions of the paper, the original preprint did not include calculated false comparisons between vaccine choice and harmful or illegal behaviour. In the revised March preprint and final publication, the following highly inappropriate material was added:

- Indirect comparisons between the choice to forgo COVID-19 vaccination with indoor cigarette smoking and driving under the influence of alcohol and other intoxicants.

- The insinuation that the unvaccinated are largely to blame for the cancellation of elective surgeries for cancer and cardiac disease, and the resulting backlogs.

- The unsubstantiated accusation that unvaccinated individuals are creating a risk that those around them may not be able to obtain the hospital care they need.

The revised versions also include references to inapplicable public health regulations that restrict freedoms in a seeming attempt to portray constitutional violations as acceptable by citing false precedent.

The inclusion of unnecessary, subjective opinions is counter to good scientific practice and has no place in what should be an objective scientific paper. The fact that CMAJ editors not only accepted these baseless and highly inflammatory remarks, but that they were inserted during the peer-review process of one of Canada's top medical journals is HIGHLY concerning.

Revision Theme #4: Stronger, More Divisive Language

The study by Fisman, Tuite and Amoako was based on a simple deterministic model that reflected the researchers' preconceived COVID-19 vaccine biases. No hypothesis was tested; hence no probability statements are possible. Any result is merely speculative, at best.

The conclusions stated in the original preprint were somewhat softer than subsequent versions — less definitive language was used and conclusions were framed as a demonstration. However, as the paper moved through the review process, the language shifted from probabilistic to deterministic, became more polarized, and implied a closer association to real-world dynamics.

As an example, compare the phrasing used in the Abstract section of the papers:

- December 16th Preprint: "While risk associated with avoiding vaccination during a virulent pandemic accrues chiefly to the unvaccinated, the choices of **these individuals <u>are likely to impact the health and safety</u>** of vaccinated individuals in a manner disproportionate to the fraction of unvaccinated individuals in the population."

- March 4th Preprint: "While risk associated with avoiding vaccination during a virulent pandemic accrues chiefly to the unvaccinated, the choices of **unvaccinated individuals <u>impact</u>** the **health and safety** of vaccinated individuals in a manner disproportionate to the fraction of unvaccinated individuals in the population."

- Published Article: "Although risk associated with avoiding vaccination during a virulent pandemic accrues chiefly **to <u>people</u> who are unvaccinated, their choices <u>affect</u> risk of viral infection** among those who are vaccinated in a manner that is disproportionate to the portion of unvaccinated **people** in the population."

In the above, the probabilistic modifier in the original claim, "likely," is dropped in the revised versions. Moreover, the nature of the impact becomes less abstract and is attributed to people, despite no people or real-world data used in the analysis. It should be noted that although the term "likely" reappears in the concluding section of all three versions, at no point in the study did the researchers demonstrate a likelihood. Any true attempt to do so would have revealed the falsity of their claims.

As another example, the revised preprint adds the concept of vaccinated people serving as a transmission "buffer" that reduces transmission rates amongst the unvaccinated when the two groups mingle. This faux benefit provided to the unvaccinated also appears in the final published version. This provably false claim is used to infer that unvaccinated people put the vaccinated at risk while reaping undeserved benefits from the vaccinated.

As a final example, the modelling demonstration presented by the researchers in the original preprint becomes a finding amongst people in the final publication:

> ... we **demonstrate** here that the choices made by **individuals** who forgo vaccination contribute (disproportionately) to risk among those who do. (December 2021 and March 2022 preprints)

> Versus

> ... we **found** that the choices made by **people** who forgo vaccination contribute disproportionately to risk among those who do get vaccinated. (Final April publication)

A demonstration can be hypothetical or theoretical whereas a finding indicates real evidence at the empirical or observational level. Moreover, it is inappropriate to attempt to pass off simulated entities as flesh-and-blood people.

A CLOSER LOOK AT CMAJ'S TOP EDITORS

Although CMAJ has an anonymous peer review process, the editor-in-chief (EiC) has full authority over the editorial content of the journal.[186] At the time of submission, Kirsten Patrick was serving as CMAJ's interim EiC. University of Toronto Professor Andreas Laupacis had vacated the position in March 2021 at which time he moved into the role as senior deputy editor of CMAJ, a position he maintained throughout the peer review process.

In the fall of 2021, interim EiC Kirsten Patrick penned an incongruent and largely unscientific opinion piece voicing strong support for vaccine mandates and passports while morally condemning those who protest such measures.[187] Throughout the piece, Kirsten made clear her belief that those who do not accept a COVID-19 vaccination threaten the health of others. The piece was published in CMAJ on October 25th, 2021.

Just over a month later, on November 29, 2021, senior deputy editor Andreas Laupacis co-authored a CMAJ article chastising physicians who refuse SARS-CoV-2 vaccination and calling for the mandatory vaccination of health care workers.[188] Like Kirsten, he believed unvaccinated staff put patients and health care colleagues at risk. Andreas' opinion appeared to stem from his misunderstanding that the novel vaccines were effective in the prevention of transmission of SARS-CoV-2. Andreas's editorial piece appeared in CMAJ just weeks before Fisman et al.'s preprint was posted online. The piece was very much in line with Fisman's messaging that vaccination cannot be considered "self-regarding" and that individual rights and freedoms are secondary to the perceived threat from unvaccinated people.

It appears that the deeply held beliefs of top CMAJ editors regarding COVID-19 vaccination may have interfered with their editorial obligations. The more one looks into this act of fraud, the clearer it becomes that CMAJ was not only complicit in the fraudulent material, they were active participants. Indeed, it seems there was a co-ordinated effort to spread disinformation throughout the medical establishment and disseminate harmful and socially destructive falsehoods to the greater community.

It is in the best interest of the medical community and all Canadians to determine the full extent of CMAJ's involvement:

- Who were all those involved in the review process?

- What were the reviewer comments?

- What role did EiC Kirsten Patrick and senior deputy editor Andreas Laupacis play?

- Who co-ordinated the media frenzy?

- Was there direct or indirect political interference with any component of the research, review process or media outreach?

These questions were put to the Ontario Provincial Police and submitted to Premier Doug Ford's office. The OPP's response is discussed in the next chapter. At the time of this writing, I had not heard back from the premier's office.

Interestingly, both Kirsten Patrick and Andreas Laupacis reaped significant rewards during and after the peer review process. In February, 2022 Kirsten Patrick was named CMAJ editor-in-chief, the first woman in the publication's history to permanently assume the role. In December 2022, Andreas Laupacis was appointed to the Order of Canada "for his ongoing contributions to the field of medicine and to a broad range of health care initiatives in Canada and around the world."[189]

University of Toronto: Deny, Deflect, Dismiss

Q: Does the University of Toronto take research integrity seriously and work to resolve all legitimate concerns as set forth in their policy guidelines?

When it came to the clear misconduct displayed by three of its researchers, the modus operandi of the University of Toronto was: deny, deflect, dismiss. As with the CMAJ correspondence, all letters and emails with the university are provided in the supplementary guide.

Letters were sent to the university's Research Oversight and Compliance Office detailing the fraudulent research and requesting an investigation of the researchers involved. The letters were addressed to Professor Lorraine E. Ferris, Associate Vice President of Research Oversight and Compliance, who acknowledged receipt of all materials and provided the university's responses to them. Three strong attempts were made to prompt the university to take action; however, they have shown extreme reluctance to look into this matter. Ultimately, U of T refused to investigate. Below is a summary of their responses to my persistent requests.

Step 1: Deny

First the oversight and compliance office denied that my complaint of research misconduct was covered under the university's Framework to Address Allegations of Research Misconduct (the "Framework"). While I had gone through the effort of providing a 20 page supporting document that detailed the misconduct, the university, in return, responded with a dismissive form letter. The paltry response claimed that the allegations specified in my complaint, including fabrication, falsification and misrepresentation of research results, did not deviate from University of Toronto norms. Certainly, if the letter is to be taken at face value, that statement speaks poorly of their research community.

Step 2: Deflect

I provided a second letter specifying the precise sections in their Framework that dealt with falsification and fabrication of data and results. In response, the university attempted to deflect from the U of T researchers' clear misconduct by misrepresenting the essence of my complaint. That is, they played dumb. The ethics officer, Professor Lori Ferris, pretended not to know the difference between what constitutes well-accepted research methodology and what constitutes a textbook case of scientific fraud.

Step 3: Dismiss

I clarified the allegations with a third letter, leaving no room for misinterpretation and eliminating any excuse for inaction. Indeed, my final letter presented a damning indictment of the university's decision not to investigate as well as one last call to adequately address the concerns and questions that I had raised. My letter ended on the following note:

Mathematical modelling does not grant one a license to mislead, to ignore real-world data, to fabricate or falsify results and call them reality. To foster such deception under the guise of science does a disservice to the scientific field, the research institute and to society.

The university responded by closing the file without addressing a single allegation or concern, despite significant effort on my part to present the issues and evidence as clearly as possible.

BOTTOM LINE: U of T Incriminates Itself

Despite the university's inaction and complete refusal to properly address and investigate two of the most serious allegations of misconduct that can be levelled against researchers, the correspondence was quite useful. In particular, the second letter written by the university showed just how weak and indefensible the research was. It's little wonder the researchers did not engage in any serious debate or open academic discussion.

The hand-waiving justifications for the poor research that were provided by the university were feeble and unbecoming of a serious academic institute. More importantly, the meager points raised in Professor Ferris's second letter provided me the opportunity to clarify the difference between useful, scientific mathematical modelling and the fictional nonsense presented by Fisman et al. Indeed, such perversion of the discipline is so foreign to most scientists in the field of mathematical modelling that it wouldn't have occurred to us that such basics would have to be spelled out.

For example, it is standard practice to validate a model and results before making inferences about real-world outcomes. David Fisman and Ashleigh Tuite surely know this since they specialize in mathematical modelling; Fisman even cites mathematical epidemiology as a primary teaching responsibility. Yet, they did not undertake any benchmarking or validation of any kind despite real-world data being readily available to test and calibrate their model and findings. It doesn't take a mathematical genius to understand that choosing to ignore inconvenient real-world trends does not give researchers a green light to replace them with ideologically favourable simulations. Just because mathematical equations were used to contrive the results doesn't make them scientific or in any way valid. The "science" being sold to the public is much different than the rigorous science of true professionals. My letters to the university are included in the supplementary reference guide, *Fisman's Fraud: the Accomplices*. The final letter to the university dispels common misconceptions in the field.

The final letter I received from the university concluded with a terse shut down of my complaint: "The University's file on this matter is closed." U of T failed to meaningfully address any of the allegations. However, the exchange successfully documented the following:

✓   Receipt of my letters requesting an investigation into the allegations of research misconduct by tenured professor David N. Fisman and two of his colleagues, Afia Amoako and Ashleigh R. Tuite.

✓   Receipt of my 20 page supporting document that articulates the many acts of scientific misconduct and fraud that were committed.

✓   The university's response to my letters, which confirm that they are aware of the work by Fisman et al. whereby the authors develop a model to simulate hypothetical COVID-19 incident rates, then attempt to pass off the results as fact.

✓   U of T's awareness that the fabricated results are contrary to real data and are being used to support discriminatory policy against those choosing not to get the COVID-19 vaccines.

✓   Awareness that the erroneous and falsified findings were widely distributed to the public through numerous media outlets, and that the fraudulent study was used in Parliament to justify extending federal travel restrictions against the unvaccinated.

✓ Awareness of data trends within Ontario and globally showing that COVID-19 (Omicron) incident rates have been disproportionately higher amongst the vaccinated, especially those boosted.

✓ Awareness that dozens of other scientists and researchers have rebuked the study by Fisman et al.; at least 22 scientists and researchers had submitted written concerns to CMAJ within the first week of its publication.

✓ Confirmation of the university's position that the conduct by David Fisman, Afia Amoako and Ashleigh R. Tuite does not deviate from the norms of their research community; and,

✓ A formal record indicating that the university has chosen not to conduct an investigation into these egregious acts, contrary to their documented Framework to Address Allegations of Research Misconduct.

CIHR: Re-Defining Fraud

Q: How did CIHR's Panel on Responsible Conduct of Research respond to a breach of policy that negatively impacted the lives of millions of Canadians?

The Tri-Agency Framework for Responsible Conduct of Research lays out the responsibilities of researchers and institutions who receive Agency funding, detailing the *minimum* requirements for addressing allegations of research misconduct. This collaborative document developed by CIHR, the Natural Sciences and Engineering Research Council (NSERC), and the Social Sciences and Humanities Research Council (SSHRC) utilizes empty assurances to convince the public that tax dollars are used responsibly. Honesty, rigor, fairness, trust, adherence to professional standards, quality, ethics... warm fuzzies abound. But is the Agency serious about these convictions?

Unfortunately, when put to the test, the panel played ignorant and, like the University of Toronto, they shirked their responsibility to the public. Purporting not to know the difference between fact and opinion, **the Agencies Presidents voted to do nothing** about the fraudulent study they funded nor the University of Toronto's failure to act in accordance with CIHR's funding agreements. Moreover, CIHR failed to correct the Parliamentary record, thus allowing the study's false claims to stand. Worse, CIHR continued to fund Dr. Fisman's deceptive hate science.[190]

CIHR's final decision read as follows:[191]

> ...allegations of breach of Agency or institutional policy are not the appropriate mechanism for addressing differences of scholarly opinion.

With more than $1 billion in expenditures each year, nearly 95% of which directly funds health research activities,[192] the Agencies Presidents appear not to know the difference between actual science and pure fiction. But are we really to believe such a facade? Let's break it down.

The Process

CIHR policy stipulates that any complaints about research misconduct must first go through the research institute where the study took place.

On June 1st, 2022, after the University of Toronto first indicated it would not be launching an investigation, CIHR was informed of the misconduct allegations against David Fisman, Ashleigh Tuite and Afia Amoako (see Letter #1 in the supplementary guide).

Once the university closed the file without adequately addressing any of the concerns, a formal complaint was sent to CIHR apprising them of University of Toronto's decision not to investigate the fraud, an apparent violation of the Tri-Agency Responsible Conduct of Research Framework (see Letter #2). CIHR was provided the full complement of supplementary material and evidence (refer to letters cc'd to CIHR as well as the full critique of the Fisman study, all provided within the supplementary guide).

Specificity of the Allegations & Impact of the Breach

The complaint against the University of Toronto included the specific policies that were breached under the Tri-Agency Framework, the severity of the violations, and the importance of addressing the misconduct allegations against the researchers. Moreover, the complaint spelled out the course of action expected of CIHR based on their proclaimed agency vision and their duties as detailed in their own policy guidelines. In order to remedy the wrongdoing I respectfully requested the following actions be taken by CIHR:

- Issue a letter of concern to the main researcher David N. Fisman.

- Request the authors retract their CMAJ publication.

- Request that the researchers make a public statement clarifying their research findings and set the record straight — that their work does not relate to real events and the main "finding" is unsupported and contrary to real-world observations.

- Notify Parliament of the fraud and inform members that the study findings presented in the House of Commons were erroneous and in fact contrary to real-world data.

- Notify all relevant public institutions and agencies of the fraud, mindful that David Fisman has served on numerous COVID-19 advisory boards and has provided legal expertise on issues related to COVID-19 epidemiology.

- Review all previous work, recommendations, and advocacy these researchers have conducted throughout the pandemic that was funded by CIHR. In particular, such work should be reviewed for errors and bias, especially in regards to COVID-19 vaccination or anything derived from mathematical modelling exercises done in part, wholly, or influenced by any of the three researchers.

- The Agency not accept applications for future funding from the researchers in relation to the COVID-19 pandemic.

The importance of setting the Parliamentary record straight was highlighted. CIHR reports to Parliament through the Minister of Health; the Deputy Minister of Health is a non-voting member of CIHR's Governing Council; and, the Parliamentary Secretary to the Minister of Health had cited the faux research in the House of Commons as an excuse to extend restrictive COVID-19 travel policies. As such, CIHR has a responsibility to inform Parliament that the research findings cited were in fact fraudulent and contrary to what had played out in Canada during the Omicron wave.

As specified in the Canadian Institutes of Health Research Act, one of the powers and functions of CIHR is to advise the Minister in respect of any matter relating to health research or health policy.[193] Surely, correcting the record of a falsity that has negatively impacted the rights and wellbeing of millions of Canadians should be given high priority.

CIHR DECISION — A Difference of Scholarly Opinion

On December 19th 2022, CIHR made a final decision with respect to the Fisman file: The Agency Presidents sided with the University of Toronto that the allegations were "differences of scholarly opinion" and, as such, they ruled that the Tri-Agency Framework for breach of policy was not the appropriate mechanism for addressing the allegations.

That ruling appears to fly in the face of the Tri-Agency's written policy — allegations of fabrication and falsification are clearly covered in the Framework. Nonetheless, CIHR closed the file and turned their backs on obvious scientific malfeasance.

It is highly concerning that the Agencies Presidents would deny knowledge of their own policies and display such lack in understanding of basic terms such as: fact, opinion, fraud, compliance, etc. Consider their word choice when describing the allegations: "scholarly opinion."

Scholarly: involving or relating to serious academic study (Cambridge dictionary); characteristic of, or suitable to learned persons (Merriam-Webster).

Opinion: A view, judgment, belief (Cambridge dictionary and Merriam-Webster).

The allegations against Fisman, Tuite and Amoako are based on fully referenced, verifiable facts. The trio fabricated and falsified results and used them to mislead the community. That is a fact, not an opinion. The researchers satisfied the literal definitions of fabrication and falsification as set out in the Tri-Agency Research Integrity Policy.

Q: What does the University of Toronto consider scholarly?

To ascertain what the University of Toronto considers scholarly, I consulted their online library and found an article entitled: "What counts as a scholarly source?"[194] The first criterion listed in the article concerns the accuracy of the information in that it should be based on **verifiable facts**. The second criterion is in regard to the **author's qualifications** and a third criterion states that there should be **no obvious bias**; the information should be based on **fact, not opinion**. The University of Toronto article also asserts that **all peer-reviewed sources are scholarly.**

So, how can the allegations against the University of Toronto researchers be considered a (mere) difference of "scholarly opinion" when, according to the university, scholarly information is based on verifiable facts and NOT biased opinions?

The fact that the "scholarly" Fisman article found its way into a peer-reviewed medical journal and has been shown to be nothing more than an overtly discriminatory and fraudulent opinion piece void of actual facts is the essence of the problem! Indeed, based on the university's own criteria of what defines a scholarly source, the publication by Fisman et al. is both scholarly (since it appeared in a peer reviewed journal) and not scholarly (since it was based on biased opinions void of facts) at the same time — a paradox! Is the university and CIHR trying to assert that the problem is itself the defense?

This is not how a serious scientific agency conducts itself. Science is rational; it is concerned with truths of the natural world. Butchering the English language to push an agenda and skirt accountability is an age-old political trick, unbecoming of research institutes.

CIHR and the University of Toronto use terms with meanings that they've specifically defined and still get them wrong. Language itself is becoming undone. How on earth are we to communicate with each other when words, even basic ones, fail to have consistent meaning?

"When I use a word," Humpty Dumpty said in rather a scornful tone, "it means just what I choose it to mean — neither more nor less."

"The question is," said Alice, "whether you can make words mean so many different things."

"The question is," said Humpty Dumpty, "which is to be master — that's all."

— Lewis Carroll, Through the Looking Glass

This game they are playing reeks of corruption and/or incompetence.

IMPLICATIONS OF THE DECISION

In essence, the federal government, through CIHR, funded fraudulent hate science, the underpinnings of which have been used as justification for discriminatory policies including travel restrictions that directly violated Charter rights and freedoms. By refusing to set the Parliamentary record straight, the Agency Presidents have shown themselves to be complicit in the deceitful activity that has been used to defraud millions of Canadians of their basic mobility rights as protected under Section 6 of the Charter. Moreover, the study's false findings, namely that the unvaccinated disproportionately contribute to risk of COVID-19 infection and transmission amongst the vaccinated population, continues to be cited as justification for the punitive restrictions that were imposed.

CIHR's decision was in complete contradiction to assurances made by Susan Zimmerman, CIHR's former executive director of the Secretariat on Responsible Conduct of Research (2007-2021). She conveyed that, as stewards of public money, CIHR is in the best position to police its researchers and ensure accuracy.[195]

> *We are interested in ensuring the public record is correct and reliable and accurate, and we are interested in fixing your conduct if you are not doing that... We are concerned if you lie on your application for funding. We are concerned if you mismanage your funds. We are concerned if, through incompetence or laziness or ignorance, you can't lay hands on accurate raw data.*

> — *Zimmerman, Executive Director of the SRCR, CIHR 2007-2021*

Did CIHR's convictions on integrity change under Zimmerman's successor, Karen Wallace, or were they always hollow?

Following their decision not to investigate the allegations of misconduct, CIHR continued to fund the bogus modelling of Fisman, Tuite and Amoako which perpetuated a provably false and harmful narrative completely detached from reality. On February 7, 2023, an updated preprint of the fraudulent study was posted online.[196] Once again the researchers used a contrived mathematical model, absent of any model validation using real-world data, to further a false notion that scapegoats individuals and promotes unsound, unconstitutional and extremely harmful policy.

In the end, all three reputable agencies — CMAJ, U of T, and CIHR — appeared content to allow a plainly fraudulent study to stand uncorrected and to continue supporting the researchers and their harmful research tactics. Clearly, something substantial was amiss. So, having exhausted the academic route, I turned to the Ontario Provincial Police for help.

CHAPTER 10

OPP: Law & Order?

Where There's No Will, There's No Way.

When dealing with the University of Toronto and CIHR's research integrity officials, it was clear they were playing dumb. Despite being well versed in standard research protocols and matters of research integrity, they stuck to the game of deny, deflect, and, when cornered, dismiss. The glaring issues with Fisman's paper, spelled out in no uncertain terms by myself and scores of other researchers, eventually reached top executives within the two organizations. They made an informed decision to stand by the fraudulent study.

Dealing with the Ontario Provincial Police (OPP) was an entirely different matter, but with similar results — inaction. When speaking with the quadruple-vaccinated OPP detective sergeant, I understood early on that convincing the OPP to conduct a proper investigation would be an uphill battle.

The Submission

Q: What, if anything, does the Anti-Rackets Branch of the Ontario Provincial Police have to offer in matters pertaining to large-scale scientific fraud?

The usual channels for dealing with research misconduct failed. I had reached out to the research institutes involved and, instead of addressing the obvious transgressions, they opted out of their responsibilities. If the influence of the researchers and their faux study had been minimal, I might have stopped there. But the stakes were too high, the societal and personal impacts too far-reaching.

So, I gathered together all my correspondences with the three institutions involved in the Fisman study and started drafting a record for the OPP. In writing the report, my goal was to do as much of the background work as possible in order to compel the OPP to do the deeper investigative work that only they have the means to accomplish. When all was said and done, I couriered a 150 page evidentiary report to the Anti-Rackets Branch of the OPP, along with a cover letter addressed to Commissioner Thomas Carrique. Additionally, I sent Premier Doug Ford's office a copy.

The material explained in detail the fraudulent activity undertaken by the researchers, its scope, and the failure of the three research institutions to investigate. I also explained why I believed the matter fell within the purview of the OPP Anti-Rackets Branch.

The Interview

On the one-year publication anniversary of the faux study, I had a phone interview with an OPP anti-rackets intake officer regarding my submission.

The 90 minute session with the detective sergeant began in a professional tone covering the nature of my complaint, the roles of the individuals and organizations involved, and how the complaint originated. We also discussed the steps I had taken to address the concerns prior to going to the OPP as well as possible next steps. While the interview was fairly cordial, signs the officer may lack the high level of professional objectivity required began to emerge.

First off, I didn't need to know his vaccination status. I didn't ask for it and it was irrelevant to the complaint at hand. The unsolicited information invited confrontation. Additionally, the officer asserting his overall satisfaction with the manner in which the pandemic was handled did little to alleviate my concerns about his ability to differentiate his personal bias from objective duty. These concerns were compounded during a second phone call when the officer disclosed that he, personally, hadn't suffered from the actions of the researchers nor from the imposed mandates. Moreover, on numerous occasions the detective steered the conversation away from the specific case at hand into vaguely specified generalizations about the overall handling of the pandemic, seeking and providing judgment on the entire COVID-19 response.

Is the importance of a complaint to the OPP measured by how the intake officer was personally impacted by the alleged misconduct? If not, why mention it?

Is this a matter for the OPP?

REGARDING FRAUD, the main questions are:

(1) Did the researchers commit a false statement? (2) Was there intent to deceive? (3) Did they obtain something of value?

The first two questions are central to the determination of research fraud. The evidence on that front is overwhelming. But, according to the detective, it is the third question that determines whether this is a matter for the OPP.

Was there a misuse of public research funds? If so, does that qualify as obtaining something of value?

Facts: The study by Fisman et al. was conducted using public funds with the main goal to "help guide Canadian health agencies as they try to control or limit the spread of COVID-19 in Canada."[197] Using those funds, the researchers simulated results contrary to real-world data and advocated for policy based on that falsity.

My viewpoint: On its surface, it appears that the funds were used to do the opposite of the intended purpose — to *mis*guide Canadian health agencies as they tried to control the spread of COVID-19. CIHR's refusal to investigate this matter indicates complicity and the need for an OPP investigation.

Was the public misled into taking an unnecessary medical treatment that directly benefits the researchers?

Facts: The main researcher, David Fisman, has been acknowledged as a highly influential figure during the pandemic. He, along with his two colleagues, used a false premise to advocate for the broad uptake of COVID-19 vaccines at a time when it was known (1) the vaccines carry a risk of serious harm, and, (2) most individuals were at very low risk of serious illness from the virus.

My viewpoint: The main researcher, David Fisman, has numerous ties to the pharmaceutical industry which seeks to benefit from his advocacy. The precise extent to which he gains personally from vaccine uptake or from his endorsement of the pharmaceuticals requires further investigation.

Could the promotion of COVID-19 vaccines and vaccine mandates, or conducting research in support of strong public health regulations, lead to career advancement or opportunities?

Facts: The Government of Canada invested heavily in university resources to promote COVID-19 vaccination and address "vaccine hesitancy." The pandemic presented opportunities in the field of epidemiology, mathematical modelling, vaccine outreach etc. For instance, Fisman's modelling work was well-funded by the federal government and he was awarded a position to lead the Centre for Pandemic Readiness in the newly created Institute for Pandemics.

My viewpoint: Given the political connections and fields of expertise of the research trio and top CMAJ editors, there is a reasonable expectation that promoting COVID-19 vaccination and providing strong support for government interventions would lead to greater career advancement and opportunities.

REGARDING PROFESSIONAL NEGLIGENCE, the main question is:

As a physician and researcher, did Fisman show a reckless disregard for the lives or safety of other persons?

Facts: Many researchers and physicians advocated for vaccine uptake without due consideration of the risks and/or whether the risks truly outweigh the benefits. Physicians were told by public health authorities that, as far as they were concerned, the vaccine benefits outweighed the risks despite a lack of evidence. Any physician saying otherwise could face strong reprimands from their medical licensing bodies.

My viewpoint: Unlike most physicians, Fisman played an influential role in informing health authorities who, in turn, dictated what other physicians could say or do regarding COVID-19 vaccination. The vaccines' ability to reduce transmission weighed into the community benefit and was a key driver in setting public policy. David Fisman and his colleagues misled the public and public health officials about this benefit.

AN OPPORTUNITY FOR RACKETEERING: During the pandemic, politicians often claimed that scientific evidence provided justification for their harsh pandemic restrictions. But if that science is shown to be both false and fraudulent, and no reasonable justification or excuse actually existed for the coercive policy, who then is accountable for the extortive tactics? Does the blame fall to the politicians who enacted the policy or to the scientist(s) who purposely misled the government? Or, is no one to be held to account for the careers that were destroyed, the financial losses that were incurred, the mental anguish and other harms the public endured for no good reason?

If the latter is the case, then the pandemic has exposed a loophole for politicians and social activists posing as researchers to use extortive tactics to circumvent an individual's freedom of choice. It seems the checks and balances are too easily manipulated. If a politician wants to justify threatening or coercive action, all they would have to do is call up a like-minded researcher/activist to get the rubber stamp. Vice-versa, a researcher/activist can provide "research" to a like-minded politician to further their cause. In the case of Fisman's fraud, key questions are:

(1) Did the researchers, on their own, have enough political or societal influence for their study to interfere with anyone's freedom of choice? (2) Did the researchers act on their own accord?

Facts: The researchers used their fraudulent research to enhance vaccine uptake by (1) advocating for coercive public policy and (2) defaming and publicly shaming unvaccinated individuals. Subsequently, the Parliamentary Secretary to the Minister of Health presented the faux study in the House of Commons to justify restrictions against the unvaccinated. Over 90 media outlets and 113 news stories circulated the country with libelous content, warning the public about the risk of mixing with the unvaccinated. Clearly, the researchers had influence.

My Viewpoint: It was well known that the federal Liberal party wanted to maintain their vaccine mandates and travel restrictions but they lacked scientific evidence for doing so. The research trio knew, or should have known, that their faux study would be used to support the coercive policies. Fisman participated in many interviews where he continued to push the false results and utter derogatory comments about the unvaccinated. By all appearances, the researchers had both political and public sway. What is not fully known is the extent to which other entities were involved. Hence the need for an OPP investigation.

Investigating a possible extortion ring is within the purview of the OPP Anti-Rackets Branch.

- There is evidence that CMAJ was actively involved in the manufacture of fraudulent statements published in the Fisman et al. report. *Did they also help orchestrate the media blitz?*

- CIHR funded the study and is ultimately responsible for informing Parliament that the research cited in the House of Commons was false. The Agency Presidents chose not to do so. On its surface, this looks incriminating. *Was there any political involvement or interference?*

Read Between the Lines

Immediately following the initial interview with the OPP, I sent a quick email to the officer summarizing the main takeaways from our call along with follow-up items. While this was the first complaint I had ever sent to the OPP, my impression of the interview was that it followed a fairly routine line of questioning to suss out the situation.

During that initial call, several indications that the OPP was reluctant to investigate surfaced and we clashed on points of law. This was not unexpected. I simply took note of the officer's comments and interpretations, let him know that I'd look into some case law to provide additional backing for my points.

The detective indicated that for an OPP investigation to occur, evidence of theft (in the narrowest sense of the word) would be needed and/or a threat of physical harm or violence (as per the detective's understanding of extortion). For matters regarding defamation, he suggested sending a complaint to the Human Rights Commission (HRC). The detective claimed to be unaware of anyone who suffered harm from the derogatory comments or vaccine mandates; he personally wasn't impacted.

For the first two of the detective's points, theft and threat, ample case law exists that refutes his narrow interpretation of the law as it pertains to possible criminal fraud or extortion. For example, threatening to post nude pictures of someone on social media unless paid would fall under extortion. The threat doesn't have to be a threat of violence. Section 346 of the Canadian Criminal Code is **broadly** worded to include blackmail, of which there have been numerous documented cases that did not involve physical harm or threat thereof.[198] Moreover, in R. v. McClure (1957),[199] the judge instructed the jury that it is up to THEM to decide whether or not the words constitute a threat. Extortion is not always about money; people have attempted to extort sexual favours, promises or tangible property.[200]

> *The level of the threats used is not as important as the intention of coercing the victim to surrender something against their will.*
>
> — *Criminal Code Help (Extortion or Blackmail Laws in Canada)*

The detective's suggestion that I take my concerns of defamation to the Ontario Human Rights Commission came off as an attempt at deflection. The commission deals with complaints of discrimination or harassment based on protected grounds in specific areas such as jobs, housing and services. The commission does not regulate hate speech; moreover, vaccination status is not currently a protected class and the commission does not deal with acts of discrimination and defamation outside its jurisdiction. It goes without saying that I ignored this dead end.

Admittedly, the detective lived insulated from the derogatory comments and discriminatory policies advocated by the researchers. He was oblivious to the suffering such actions might have caused others. I suggested he view some of the first-hand testimony coming out of the National Citizen's Inquiry (NCI) that was taking place at the time. I also informed him that he had just spent over an hour speaking with someone whose entire family had suffered resultant harm.

I arranged to get back to the detective the next week for a follow on conversation to address his comments. In the meantime, I delved into case law and engaged in long conversations with individuals in the legal profession. However, despite my efforts, in the hours leading up to our planned discussion a decision already had been made. There would be no investigation.

Cognitive Dissonance: "Everyone's Doing It"

The follow-up phone conversation did not go as anticipated. For the most part, I was unable to get through the additional material I had gathered — the detective cut me off, informing me the matter would not be pursued.

I tried to home in on the reasoning for the OPP's decision and get an idea of how far up the chain of command my complaint had gone. And although the detective assured me the complaint had risen to higher levels, he would only provide me with the name and email address of his immediate supervisor. My attempts to get to the bottom of the OPP's decision-making specifics appeared to agitate him. Instead of narrowing the scope, he blew it wide open: *"Don't you think the government did the best they could? The whole world acted the same way…"*

No. I don't think the government did the best they could, nor do I think they had the public's best interests at heart. But that's beside the point. I explained to the detective that I wasn't asking the OPP to investigate the government's entire pandemic response. My goal was to draw attention to a rather simple and provable act of misconduct that has had, and continues to have, huge societal implications. Even if one agreed with the way the pandemic was handled in every respect, it's still not acceptable for a research team to deceive the public and to demonize a segment of society.

But the quad-vaxxed detective did not see the harms done. He made it clear that his myopic interpretation of the law was not up for discussion. I tried to convey the importance of collecting the facts and not allowing one person's subjective views to override the interests of millions of Canadians — that it is not up to either one of us to play judge and jury. From the comments that followed, I got the impression that he didn't see his interpretation of the law as a mere opinion.

The detective hadn't taken up my earlier suggestion to watch the testimonies from the National Citizen's Inquiry either. He put aside the first-hand accounts of the massive suffering that took place. Uninterested, I suppose.

Implications

My initial letter to the OPP contained the following excerpt with regards to the inaction of CMAJ, the University of Toronto and CIHR to investigate the faux study:

> *Each of the three organizations have a demonstrated conflict of interest in investigating this matter and have instead opted to ignore the indisputable facts. When establishments tasked with protecting society against such malicious acts relent on their duty in favour of self-interests, there are grave*

consequences to the health and well-being of citizens. Providing cover for overt and irrefutable fraud not only undermines public trust in our institutions, it allows the resultant harm caused by the fraud to propagate. These acts of complicity are deeply troubling. It is paramount that an independent policing agency look into this matter to ensure the public's interests are served, to prevent further harm from accruing, and to protect the public from any related racketeering activities or efforts.

While I had hoped the OPP would take this to heart, I had been cautioned about that unlikelihood. A local OPP officer had looked over my report and offered suggestions on what type of material to include prior to my formal submission. He had been the one to suggest that I send it to the Anti-Rackets Branch, given its scope and importance. While I have no doubt he was very interested in the report and also hoped it would gain traction, he cautioned the odds weren't good. Given what he'd seen from the force and their dismissive attitude towards anyone who had voiced concerns about how the pandemic was handled, he figured maybe 1 officer out of 100 would care enough to do something. Another OPP officer that I spoke with, this one retired, thought those odds were optimistic. He didn't believe there was a chance in hell the OPP would investigate a case that exposed fraud on such a topic, no matter what evidence was presented — "they're too invested in the vaccine narrative," he cautioned.

So, I knew full well that my submission was a long shot. But, by filing the complaint, at least it would go on record — the best I could hope for.

CHAPTER 11

The Need for Protected Status

When researchers are willing to commit fraud to scapegoat a vulnerable group, health agencies willing to promote it, academic institutions ready to defend it, and the government eager to fund it, then that group needs protected status.

It is clear that individuals who chose to forgo COVID-19 vaccination have been targeted with extreme hostility to restrict their civil liberties without due justification and, in the current instance, through fraudulent means.

Fisman's fraud was funded by the Government of Canada, supported by the University of Toronto, and disseminated to the public by the Canadian Medical Association Journal as well as numerous national and international media outlets. Moreover, CMAJ appears to have played an active role in the crafting of the fraudulent hate science. The university rewarded two of the fraudulent modellers with top roles in a new Institute for Pandemics and CIHR continued to fund updates of the bogus modelling in order to keep the false narrative alive.

The three institutes ignored their own public mission statements regarding their commitment to improved health for Canadians and best practices in research. Furthermore, governance councils seemed to have applied contrary meanings for honesty and integrity from what appears in their policy documents.

While much of this book focused on the contents of the hate science piece authored by the University of Toronto trio, its general acceptance signifies a much deeper problem than this single fraudulent study. There is simply too much readily available and irrefutable evidence about the non-sterilizing nature of the COVID-19 vaccines and their inability to curb transmission for such scapegoating tactics to survive academia without outside influence. As discussed in Chapter 6, politics has been a key driver in the faux narrative.

Politics Dictating Science

The vaccines' failure to curb transmission became apparent in the early days of the Delta variant with numerous outbreaks reported in venues with highly vaccinated populations. By early August 2021, CDC had analyzed the infection data stemming from the large Massachusetts outbreak the month prior. The vast majority of cases were amongst the fully vaccinated (74%), the average time since their second vaccine dose was just under 3 months and the viral loads of fully vaccinated cases were similar to those of unvaccinated or partially vaccinated cases.[201]

By the fall of 2021 several international journal articles had already been written regarding the vaccines' failure to curtail community transmission. Subramanian and Kumar (2021) found that increases in COVID-19 were unrelated to levels of vaccination across 68 countries and 2947 counties in the United States.[202]

Acharya et al (2022) found that viral loads from nasal swabs were similar among unvaccinated and vaccinated individuals infected with the SARS-CoV-2 delta variant.[203]

Bardosh et al. (2022) aptly pointed out that these transmission trends had been painfully obvious to anyone paying attention:

> *Since early reports of post-vaccination transmission in mid-2021, **it has become clear** that vaccinated and unvaccinated individuals, once infected, transmit to others at similar rates.*

> — *Bardosh et al. (BMJ Global Health 2022)*[204]

Indeed, this was all known *before* the federal government imposed its vaccine mandates and the provinces implemented their vaccine passports, as discussed in Chapter 6. Then, in the early days of the Omicron outbreak, infection rate data from highly vaccinated countries such as Denmark and the United Kingdom showed *higher* infection rates amongst the fully vaccinated compared to those who were unvaccinated.[205] That is, the higher rates of infection amongst the vaccinated were not unique to Ontario. It was happening globally. So how could Fisman's easily disproven study have gotten so much traction in Canada?

The government and all those who supported the hate, discrimination and human rights violations that went with vaccine mandates and passports were in desperate need of scientific evidence to justify the unjustifiable. Fisman and his colleagues fulfilled that need with an eye to the future.

Purposeful Division

The tactics used in Fisman's paper — scapegoating, shaming using pejorative terms, promoting discrimination and human rights violations as a means to increase vaccination — have been the go-to tactics embraced by politicians and top public health authorities throughout the pandemic. Such transgressions were not spurred by evidence or societal good. On the contrary. The point of vaccine passports and restrictions was, as President Macron crudely stated, to make life miserable for the unvaccinated. Consider his words as Omicron whipped through France's mostly vaccinated population:[206]

> *I really want to piss them [the unvaccinated] off. And so we're going to keep on doing it, until the end. That's the strategy.*

> — *President Emmanuel Macron, January 4, 2022*

That was the strategy — to "piss off" the unvaccinated; to make their lives as unbearable as possible so that they'd finally surrender to the will of the politicians and take the injection. Days later, the French parliament voted to introduce the vaccine passport to do just that. By that time, Canadian provinces were already several months into their vaccine passport systems. While countries such as France and Canada were suffocating their populace with additional restrictions, other countries eyed the post-vaccination COVID-19 surge with some degree of self-reflection. There were growing calls in Europe for the coronavirus to be treated like other transmissible illnesses such as the flu.[207] PM Boris Johnson announced the end of all COVID-related restrictions in England. The United States Supreme Court blocked President Biden's workplace vaccine mandate.

PM Trudeau, however, appeared to be emboldened by the French President's remarks and ramped up his own rhetoric against the unvaccinated. A day after Macron vowed to "piss off" the unvaccinated, PM Trudeau was calling them "anti-vaxxers" (once again) and blamed them for the latest round of government-imposed lockdowns.[208] At the time, Canadian provinces were experiencing some of the harshest lockdowns in the world.[209] Quebec, for example, had gone so far as to impose a curfew and prescribe fines of up to $6,000 for anyone outside their home after 10 p.m. Other provinces searched for additional penalties and restrictions to impose on the unvaccinated, above the ones that had already been in place for months. New Brunswick Premier Blaine Higgs openly pledged to make the lives of the unvaccinated "increasingly uncomfortable" and looked to Quebec for pointers — the francophone province had recently witnessed an uptake in first-dose vaccinations after adding liquor and cannabis stores to the list of venues requiring a COVID-19 vaccine passport.[210] Quebec Premier Legault threatened to go even farther and impose a health tax on the unvaccinated.[211]

The highly effective political tactic of scapegoating had been embraced by the federal Liberal government early into the vaccine rollout. According to Liberal MP Joël Lightbound, his party made the decision to vilify the unvaccinated on the eve of the 2021 federal election campaign. They were hoping the societal wedge would catapult them to a majority government.

A decision was made to wedge, to divide and to stigmatize.

— Liberal MP Joël Lightbound on the Liberal 2021 election campaign[212]

In mid-August 2021, the Trudeau government announced their plans to require COVID-19 vaccination of the federal workforce and the federally regulated transportation sector.[213] Two days later, the 2021 federal election was officially announced. With approximately 72% of the eligible population fully vaccinated and 82% with at least one dose, Trudeau spent the first day of the campaign pitting the vaccinated majority against the unvaccinated minority, blaming them for disease transmission.[214] He and his government continued to push that divide further and further with increased vehemence and mounting threats. During campaign stops he assured the masses that his government was protecting society against the danger posed by the wrong-thinking "anti-vaxxers" who were putting kids, families and others at risk.[215]

> *The anti-vaxxers, they're wrong. They're wrong about how we get through this pandemic. And more than just being wrong, 'cause everyone's entitled to their opinions, they are putting at risk their own kids, and they are putting at risk our kids as well. That's why we've been unequivocal. If you want to get on a plane or train in the coming months you're going to have to be fully vaccinated so that families with their kids don't have to worry that someone is going to put them in danger in the seat next to them or across the aisle.*

> —*Prime Minister Justin Trudeau, August 31, 2021*

No evidence was ever provided that such exclusionary policies were needed, effective or anything other than political in nature.

In the days and months that followed, an endless stream of unsubstantiated claims vilifying the unvaccinated as disease spreaders were used to unite the majority and rally support for discriminatory policies. Provinces were encouraged to get on board and develop vaccine passports, the promise of federal funding dangling like a carrot on a stick. [216] Rhetoric against the unvaccinated reached dangerous levels. Open hostility, vitriol and misinformation spewed from the highest levels of government, seeping into public opinion and fueling societal divide. Media outlets capitalized on the hate and ran with sensationalized headlines (see Figure 12).

Canada had entered into a truly dark period. PM Trudeau's shocking remarks in a French-language TV interview during his election campaign illustrate the country's downward spiral:[217]

> *Yes, we will emerge from this pandemic through vaccination. We know people*

who are still making up their minds and we will try to convince them, but there are also people who are vehemently opposed to vaccination. They do not believe in science, who are often misogynists, often racists, too; it is a sect, a small group, but who are taking up space, and here we have to make a choice, as a leader, as a country. Do we tolerate these people?

— *Prime Minister Justin Trudeau, September 2021 (translated from French)*

"Do we tolerate these people?" — an eerie sentiment inflicted upon millions of unvaccinated Canadians. Trudeau had warned that there would be "consequences"[218] if certain individuals chose not to get fully vaccinated. That warning was followed by threats (promises) of stripping them of mobility rights and cutting off the employment income of those unvaccinated who worked for the federal government. While the Liberals fell very short of a majority, it didn't much matter. They won a minority government and struck an agreement with the socialist NDP party who basically gave them carte blanche.[219]

Upon re-election, the prime minister followed through with his threats and went a step further. The Government of Canada updated their guidelines to exclude the unvaccinated from collecting Employment Insurance.[220] That is, individuals terminated or put on leave without pay for not complying with a vaccination mandate (imposed by any employer, federal or otherwise) faced denial of the temporary income support they'd paid into. Desperate for work, many tried to find alternative employment during a period when businesses were being openly encouraged to ban the unvaccinated, and nearly all new jobs were in the public sector.[221] How can such cruelty be for the public good?

The Liberal government had wedged its way into the daily lives of millions of Canadians, its destructive policies destroyed dreams, careers, relationships and health. My family was among the millions of Canadians who suffered irreparable harm from the vindictive policies and the cartel of so-called experts who callously supported them. But Omicron refused to play ball. No amount of statistical manipulation could twist the data in a direction that supported the mass discrimination against the unvaccinated. With the disease-spreading anti-vaxxer narrative crumbling, Fisman, Tuite and Amoako sought to legitimize and reinforce the stigma through pure data fabrication.

Figure 12: Toronto Star, Front Page August 26, 2021

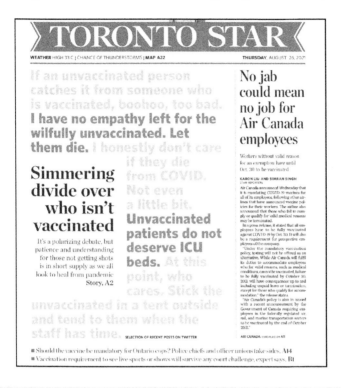

In August 2021, the Toronto Star, Canada's largest daily print newspaper, ran a front page collage of inflammatory comments accompanied by an article about the growing disdain for the unvaccinated.[222] A sample of the large bold type on the front page included: *"I have no empathy left for the willfully unvaccinated. Let them die."* and *"Unvaccinated COVID-19 patients do not deserve ICU beds."* After receiving immense backlash, the Star issued a hollow retraction. Referring to the unvaccinated as "anti-vaxxers" and painting them as selfish trouble-makers willfully putting others at risk became a recurring theme for the Toronto Star and other corporate news outlets in the months that followed.[223]

The document by Koen Swinkles, "A History of the Persecution of the Unvaccinated in COVID Era Canada (2022)," provides an in-depth examination of the hate directed against the unvaccinated during this dark period in Canadian history.

The Canadian government advocated for a two-tiered segregated social system, pretending it had scientific basis. The University of Toronto trio, led by Fisman, attempted to give them the needed "evidence." In fact, it was fraudulent hate science, unethical and socially harmful.

Fisman and his two colleagues perpetuated the false notion that COVID-19 vaccination reduces transmission — that in and of itself is potentially harmful. But they went much further. Void of any pertinent analysis or consideration, the trio advocated for punitive public health policies to coerce individuals to accept (additional) vaccine doses. They did so with complete disregard of the many harms likely to be incurred from such tactics.

The study by Bardosh et al. (2022) laid bare the damaging effects that COVID-19 vaccine mandates, passports, and restrictions have had on public trust, vaccine confidence, political polarization, human rights, inequities, and social wellbeing. They concluded that the mandatory COVID-19 vaccine policies were "scientifically questionable and are likely to cause more societal harm than good." The authors reached that verdict based on the immense harm likely to arise from these policies. They did so without having to delve into the *additional* physical and psychological harms that accrue from serious vaccine adverse events, and without any consideration of the potential role the leaky vaccines have played in driving variants and future infectivity.

But, as demonstrated throughout this book, Fisman, Tuite, Amoako, CMAJ, University of Toronto and CIHR all have stood staunchly behind the faux narrative and appear to be impervious to fact, reason or any research that invalidates their ill-conceived claims. It seems no amount of evidence will get in the way of the powerful anti-science engine fuelling their convictions. The enormous harms stemming from the government's coercive measures continue to be ignored. Public funds are still being used to normalize stigma against people who remain unvaccinated.

Fear, unfounded blame and fraudulent science were used to legitimize the discrimination of the unvaccinated. With the advent of vaccine passports, this group became identifiable and was subjected to inhumane treatment and ongoing discrimination. There is a clear need for provinces to amend their Human Rights Codes & Acts by making vaccination status a protected ground against discrimination.

Establishing a Fail-Safe: The Human Rights Code

The federally-backed vaccine passport system demanded that Canadians age twelve and older take an experimental injection in order to partake in society. This was done without demonstrated need or proof of benefit.

Regarding the need, from the very start of the pandemic COVID-19 was known to be a disease that mostly affected the very elderly and those with underlying health conditions. By May of 2020, the CDC had estimated the survival rate to be around 99.7%.[224] For those under the age of 70 yrs, estimates were in the range of 99.95% (Ioannidis, 2020).[225]

Regarding the benefit, many studies indicate that the excessive harm stemming from COVID-19 vaccine mandates and restrictions have outweighed any perceived benefits. Policies aimed at restricting unvaccinated individuals from public venues and places of employment were mostly based on hand-waiving heuristics, void of scientific evidence.

If the government can mandate a vaccine against a disease with such a high survival rate, one that poses little threat to the vast majority of individuals, they can do it for anything — unless protections are put in place.

The Canadian Human Rights Act (CHRA, the "Act") protects people in Canada from certain types of discriminatory practices when they are employed by or receive services from the federal government, First Nations governments or private companies that are regulated by the federal government.[226] More specifically, Canadians are protected from discriminatory practices based on prohibited grounds as specified in the Act:[227]

> 3 (1) For all purposes of this Act, the prohibited grounds of discrimination are race, national or ethnic origin, colour, religion, age, sex, sexual orientation, gender identity or expression, marital status, family status, genetic characteristics, disability and conviction for an offence for which a pardon has been granted or in respect of which a record suspension has been ordered.

Provincial and territorial human rights laws are very similar to the CHRA. They protect people from discrimination in areas of provincial and territorial jurisdiction, such as restaurants, stores, schools, housing and most workplaces.

Currently, vaccination status is not a prohibited ground of discrimination. Indeed, the need for such a designation was largely unforeseen since the notion of vaccine passports was unfathomable in Canada prior to 2021. Moreover, prior to the pandemic vaccine mandates were considered unconstitutional.

When the passports were first rolled out, the British Columbia Office of the Human Rights Commissioner issued the following statement:

> *No one should experience harassment or unjustifiable discrimination for not being immunized when there are effective alternatives to vaccination status policies.*
>
> *—BC Office of the Human Rights Commissioner, October 2021*[228]

Regardless of how provincial human rights commissions felt about harassment or discrimination based on vaccination status, they appeared unwilling to do anything about it. Instead, they claimed it was outside their purview. Generally speaking, provincial human rights commissions do not have the jurisdiction to prohibit discrimination outside the protected grounds as specified in their codes. The Alberta Human Rights Commission made this clear:[229]

> *Under Alberta's human rights legislation, the Commission has no jurisdiction to address claims that mandatory vaccine policies violated rights on the basis of personal opinion or political beliefs. The Commission also cannot address claims of rights violations under the Charter or other legislation, codes or acts....*
>
> *The Commission cannot accept complaints of rights violations under the Charter or any other legislation, on the basis of personal opinion or political beliefs, or any other basis not covered under the Alberta Human Rights Act at the time of any incident of discrimination.*
>
> *— Alberta Human Rights Commission, December 2022*

Provincial Human Rights Codes don't have jurisdiction outside the prohibited grounds of discrimination as specified in their codes.

Some individuals tried to avoid COVID-19 vaccination and the discrimination that comes with that choice by applying for a vaccine exemption. Two grounds protected by the CHRA and the provincial codes offered potential avenues for exemption: religious basis or medical reasons. With regard to religion or creed, the following statement by the Newfoundland & Labrador Human Rights Commission was fairly representative of the views across the various commissions:

> *The Commission is not aware of any major religion having a theological opposition to vaccines.*
>
> *— Nfld & Labrador Human Rights Commission[230]*

As such, exemptions based on religious grounds were often disputed while vaccine accommodations based on creed were generally dismissed. Creed arguments were often belittled, equated to personal preferences unconnected to any core value or belief system. Preferences are not grounds for exemption.

In terms of vaccine exemptions based on disability or medical grounds, very few medical conditions were considered eligible for such an exemption.

> *Very rarely a person may need to delay vaccination because of severe allergies, illness or severe reaction after the first dose.*
>
> *— BC Center for Disease Control, Updated December 29, 2022[231]*

Because vaccination is not specified as a prohibited ground of discrimination, unvaccinated Canadians could not turn to the human rights commissions for protection against the egregious acts of hate and discrimination that they were facing. Instead of protecting Canadians from discrimination, the constraints within the provincial codes were used to bolster the government's position.

The provincial commissions develop policies to prevent discrimination based on designated factors, of which vaccination is not one. Thus, the commissions, by and large, took the position that vaccine policies were not discriminatory with respect to the human rights codes if all persons across the designated groups had equal access to COVID-19 vaccination. That is, so long as everyone had equal opportunity to have their right to bodily autonomy violated in order to avoid discrimination, the vaccine policies were deemed compliant with the Human Rights Act and the provincial codes.

So, instead of protecting Canadians against harm and societal division caused by vaccine passports and mandates, the Human Rights Act and the provincial codes helped the government ensure that the genetic vaccines were readily available to force into everyone. This aligned perfectly with the government's vaccine agenda to have every eligible Canadian vaccinated.

The Human Rights Act and provincial codes need to be amended to include vaccine choice as a prohibited ground of discrimination. Currently, there is a huge gap in human rights protections with demonstrated potential for government exploitation.

The need for such an amendment has been recognized by Alberta Premier Danielle Smith. In an October 2022 news conference, Smith acknowledged the extreme discrimination that had been faced by unvaccinated Canadians.[232]

> *They (unvaccinated) have been the most discriminated against group that I've ever witnessed in my lifetime. That's a pretty extreme level of discrimination that we have seen.*
>
> — *Alberta Premier Danielle Smith, October 2022*

Smith went on to say that the discrimination was unacceptable and that her government would not be creating a segregated society on the basis of a medical choice. She added that the best way to counter the discrimination is to amend the Alberta Human Rights Act to add vaccination status as a grounds subject to protection from discrimination.

While vaccination status is not explicitly stated as protected grounds in the Canadian and provincial human rights codes, the interpretation that discrimination based on vaccination status does not violate the codes is logically flawed. Consider the statement made by the Ontario Human Rights Commission:[233]

> Under the Human Rights Code, an employer may not discipline or terminate an employee who has been diagnosed with COVID-19 or is perceived to have COVID-19 (because, for example, they are exhibiting certain symptoms). Similarly, an employer may not discipline or terminate an employee if they are unable to come to work because medical or health officials have quarantined them or have advised them to self-isolate and stay home in connection with COVID-19.

Here we have a situation where employees who actually have a transmissible disease cannot be disciplined or terminated by their employer, but employees who are perceived to be at greater risk of one day catching the disease can be disciplined based on that potential future situation. This reasoning presents a huge logical flaw in both disease management and human rights protections. It's shown to be even more illogical when one considers that known risk factors — like age, which changes the risk profile of the disease a thousand fold — are ignored because those factors are explicitly protected under the codes. Indeed, the top two known risk factors for COVID-19 severity, age and comorbid disabilities, are both protected grounds for discrimination.

The interpretation that discrimination based on vaccination status isn't in violation of the Canadian Human Rights Act and the provincial codes represents a logical fallacy.

CHAPTER 12

One by One They all Fell Down

"The history of liberty has largely been the history of the observance of procedural safeguards."
— *Felix Frankfurter, American Judge (1882–1965)*

Fundamental principles provide a strong foundation that supports rational decision-making, especially during times of emergency. New techniques and procedures can develop from fundamental building blocks to handle unexpected challenges. Abandoning the basics for a quick-fix often leads to failure and disappointment.

During the pandemic, governing bodies surrendered fundamental practices in science, health care, democratic governance and law. One by one, all the safeguards that had been built up over decades were abandoned. The cost to liberty and societal well-being has been devastating.

While most COVID-related restrictions and vaccine mandates have been suspended for the moment, there have been a number of holdouts (such as the public health care vaccine mandates in BC still in effect as of July 2023) and there are concerns that one day the blanket measures will resurface.[234]

Q: What is the likelihood vaccine mandates or passports will re-appear in the future?

To help answer that question, it is instructive to identify key systemwide failures that enabled their implementation.

The massive uptake of COVID-19 vaccinations was predicated on the government's ability to successfully and systematically dismantle safeguards within Canada's drug approval process and the laws that protect an individual from unnecessary and unwanted medical intrusions. The ultimate failure of our legal system to uphold Charter rights and freedoms has brought Canadian democracy to a tipping point. Attempts are being made to reinterpret fundamentals and bastardize democracy in much the same vein science has been bastardized throughout the pandemic. Indeed, faux pandemic science has been used to further this societal degradation. It was in this capacity that the idea behind Fisman's study was first conceived. Its main purpose: the dismantling of our last line of defense — the right to bodily autonomy and the ability to say "no" to government intrusion of our physical selves.

Safeguard Failure #1: Clinical Trial Protocols

> **The clinical trials were not designed to ensure safety nor to detect a reduction in any serious outcome. They were designed for superficial success.**

The human body is a complex biological system. It is impossible to anticipate all the potential health effects resulting from the multiple, interacting biological mechanisms at play when introducing a novel pharmaceutical. In theory, new genetic vaccines could offer protections, but many theoretical pathways lead to harm. That is why theory must be followed by thorough experimentation before putting any drug on the market. The theoretical benefits must be put to the test, serious adverse effects identified, and the risks quantified to ensure safety and overall health benefit.

A pharmaceutical is of little use if it alleviates one ailment only to cause another of equal or greater concern. Thus, it is important that primary endpoints of a clinical trial are clinically relevant and provide an adequate assessment of the efficacy and safety of the drug being studied. Unfortunately, the clinical trials for the COVID-19 vaccines were not designed to assess outcomes of key interest to the public, nor were they designed to map out a full safety profile. Inadequate sample sizes, short observational periods, limited safety measurements, clinically irrelevant measures of vaccine efficacy, questionable methodology, breaches in protocol (such as unblinding) are just a few of the trials' many shortcomings.

In the end, the clinical trial experiments did not establish a reduction in endpoints of key interest: transmission, all-cause hospitalization or all-cause mortality.[235] The following expert statement submitted to the European General Court in regards to EU's authorization of the use of Pfizer's mRNA vaccine on children of 12 years and older sums this up perfectly. The quoted experts note that while their arguments specifically reference the Pfizer vaccine, they apply similarly to the Moderna mRNA vaccine, and many also apply to the adenovector-based AstraZeneca and Johnson & Johnson (Janssen) vaccines.[236]

Statement of Reality:

"The clinical trials carried out by Pfizer contain no proof of any benefit conferred by the vaccine with respect to any clinically relevant endpoints. This applies to all tested age groups, and in particular also to adolescents."
— *M. Palmer MD, S. Bhakdi MD, S. Hockertz PhD*

(and pretty much anyone who actually read and understood the clinical trial reports)

And it goes downhill from there since the "efficacy" of these vaccines against variants only gets worse.

In terms of assessing safety, numerous deficiencies in the preclinical phase were evident, including: a lack of genotoxicity and drug interaction studies; tiny sample sizes for the limited safety tests that were completed; and, lack of follow-up regarding preclinical indications of potential harm (Palmer et al., 2021).[237] The shortcomings didn't end there. Phase 2/3 (phases 2 and 3 combined) of the clinical trials were very limited in the safety measurements taken, mostly relying on descriptive self-assessments rather than quantitative diagnostic tests. As such, a number of adverse events and subclinical manifestations likely went undetected. Moreover, the approximate two month observational window used for the primary analysis of the clinical trials was far too short to assess mid or long-term safety.

The clinical trial experiments did not establish that COVID-19 vaccines were "safe and effective" in any meaningful sense.

Despite major limitations with these studies, statistically significant indications of safety issues were observed. As discussed in Fraiman et al. (Vaccine, 2022), the Pfizer and Moderna mRNA COVID-19 vaccines were associated with an excess risk of serious adverse events of special interest.

Safeguard Failure #2: Drug Approval & Procurement

Standard drug approval protocols were circumvented for COVID-19 vaccines to allow for quick approval and premature uptake.

Standard research protocol puts the onus of proving the safety and efficacy of a drug on the pharmaceutical company. They collect the data. They control the data. We, the consumers, do not.

Health Canada was obligated to ensure that proper testing had been undertaken and standard scientific protocols followed. Instead, the agency side-stepped the established drug approval process, spurred on by the perceived urgency of the pandemic. On December 9, 2020, Health Canada issued the following statement:[238]

Health Canada received Pfizer's submission on October 9, 2020 and after a thorough, independent review of the evidence, Health Canada has determined that the Pfizer-BioNTech vaccine meets the Department's stringent safety, efficacy and quality requirements for use in Canada.

In reality, the vaccine was approved based on scant preliminary findings with no mid or long-term safety data whatsoever, no proof of efficacy in regards to key clinically relevant endpoints, and without the necessary monitoring in place to ensure quality of the product.[239] The vaccines were very much in the experimental phase of development and in the true sense of the word: key safety and efficacy outcomes were either untested, not yet established or not yet finalized. It is inconsistent for public health authorities to claim the vaccines were not experimental at the time of authorization while, in the same breath, claim the injections reduce hospitalization and death when these outcomes had not been established.

Shocking testimony at the NCI by Shawn Buckley, a constitutional lawyer specializing in the food and drug act, revealed the lack of safety and efficacy requirements for the approval of COVID-19 vaccines in Canada.[240] In essence, according to the testimony, Health Canada re-wrote their guidelines, basically giving COVID-19 vaccines a free pass when it came to proving safety, efficacy or conducting a proper risk-benefit assessment.

Instead of being truthful with Canadians about the preliminary state of COVID-19 vaccine research and the many uncertainties regarding safety and efficacy, government officials misled the public with false assurances. And instead of taking a cautious approach to introducing a new drug and offering it to people at most risk from the virus, federal and provincial governments demanded the entire population roll up their sleeves despite little possible benefit for the vast majority. They made no allowances for being wrong. No contingency. They showed complete recklessness and disregard for the health and safety of Canadians.

Key theoretical benefits were not established, nor realized, before the new genetic vaccines were administered into the arms of millions of Canadians.

Within a year, COVID-19 vaccines went from interim approval to full approval.[241] As Shawn Buckley explained during his NCI testimony, this was not because the drugs finally completed the standard drug approval process and necessary testing, but because the lax criteria used for interim approval of COVID-19 vaccines were silently incorporated into the regular approval process.

The government disregarded well-established scientific methodology and bi-passed their usual, more stringent requirements for drug approval. Furthermore, deceptive language was used to assure Canadians that the genetic vaccines were safe and effective — a claim they never had to back legally nor scientifically.

COVID-19 procurement contracts with the pharmaceutical companies were signed under a shroud of secrecy.

Copies of the COVID-19 procurement contracts available for parliamentary scrutiny were subjected to an unprecedented level of redactions — about fifty times that of other vaccine contracts. The Liberal government informed members of Parliament that if they wanted to see unredacted contracts they'd have to sign non-disclosure agreements (NDAs).

During a House of Commons meeting in February 2023, Liberal MP Anthony Housefather admitted that vaccine production had been rushed, the normal amount of testing hadn't been done on the products and that the contacts sought to protect the companies from liability.[242]

> *These agreements require employees of the Government of Canada who access these documents to sign confidentiality agreements.*
>
> *Why is that? Why are there many more redactions, as my colleague said, in these documents than in other documents? It's because these documents were signed at the beginning of the pandemic, when everybody was desperate for vaccines. Companies were being told to rush vaccine production and do testing in an unprecedented way, in a way that they don't normally do it.*
>
> *These companies were exposed to a way higher liability in putting their products on the market than they normally would be, because they didn't do the type of testing that normally means these drugs take years to come to market. They did it all in less than a year.*

> *That's why these companies said that if they were going to deliver this product that they hadn't tested in their normal way, they wanted to have different conditions.*
>
> — *MP Housefather, House of Commons, February 13, 2023*

In other words, the Liberal government felt it was perfectly justified to, essentially, transfer the liability from powerful pharmaceutical companies to average Canadian consumers. Drug companies were guaranteed massive sales and record-breaking profits with zero liability while Canadians were handed empty assurances and moral platitudes about "doing the right thing."

During the House of Commons meeting, opposition MP Nathalie Sinclair-Desgagné accused the Liberal MP of being "a proud representative of pharmaceutical companies." Indeed, throughout the pandemic *many* government officials had acted more like pharmaceutical salespersons than public servants — having purchased such vast amounts of the vaccine, it's no wonder. The premature and secretive procurement of hundreds of millions of doses of a novel drug put high-ranking government officials in a massive conflict of interest.

It is under this lens that government tactics should be viewed.

Consider the strong claims made by officials regarding the COVID-19 vaccines' safety and their ability to reduce transmission, severe illness and death — none of which were scientifically established. According to Health Canada, advertising or promoting drugs using false, deceptive or misleading claims is prohibited in Canada.[243] Moreover, pharmaceutical companies who promote their product by exaggerating their effectiveness, or by omitting or downplaying risks, can face **criminal charges for illegal marketing practices**.[244] Of course, pharmaceutical companies had little need to engage in such untoward practices during the pandemic since many top government officials, health care professionals, and researchers (such as Fisman and his colleagues) were more than willing to take on the task.

Safeguard Failure #3: Post-Market Surveillance

No active surveillance systems were put in place to adequately track adverse vaccine events.

In the original mRNA clinical trial protocols, study participants were to be followed for two years after their second dose. Instead, placebo recipients were offered the vaccine after completing 6 months of follow-up.[245] This "unblinding" of the clinical trials eradicated the control groups, thus thwarting any rigorous assessment of long-term safety.

The unblinding of the clinical trials made post-market surveillance all the more important. Yet, the vaccines were put on the market with no active surveillance systems in place to adequately track adverse vaccine events.[246] To a large extent, the ability to accurately assess mid or long-term adverse health risks either caused or exacerbated by the new genetic vaccines has been lost. While prospective, reasonably controlled studies could have been undertaken to examine some of the more serious adverse events that were flagged during the vaccines' rollout, Canadian health agencies and research institutes showed little interest in conducting them.

With regards to monitoring effectiveness, public health authorities adopted the use of observational data and unreliable statistics such as COVID-19 cases, COVID-19 hospitalizations and COVID-19 deaths to estimate (and inflate) vaccine benefit. As discussed in Chapter 5, observational data are fraught with confounding issues and selection biases while COVID-specific metrics are subject to substantial misclassification and reliability issues. They are also inherently biased in favour of vaccination.

Consider, for example, the difference between using all-cause mortality versus COVID-19 deaths. The former captures both the intended as well as any unintended impacts of the new vaccines on mortality. COVID-19 deaths, on the other hand, may capture the impact of the vaccine on deaths attributable to the SARS-CoV-2 virus, but that may be of little consolation if the vaccine increases the chance of dying from something else. Moreover, attributing a death or hospitalization to COVID-19 is, in itself, highly problematic since well-over 90% of such cases in Canada have had at least one underlying comorbid condition.[247] CDC has reported that 95% of COVID-19 related deaths in the USA to June 18, 2023 had additional conditions mentioned on their death certificates; these deaths had, on average, four additional health concerns.[248]

In short, authorities are not collecting the data required to scientifically prove their assertions regarding the vaccines' ability to reduce hospitalization, severe illness and death. Nor are they doing the surveillance necessary to assess safety to within a reasonable degree of confidence. Instead of following through on activities that would produce stronger, more conclusive evidence of safety and net benefit, massive resources have been directed towards activities that ensure the vaccines are *perceived* as safe and effective. The emphasis has always been on enhancing vaccine uptake as opposed to actual health and safety.

The cost associated with proper post-market follow-up doesn't appear to be the main factor for the lack of interest. Certainly, the pharmaceutical companies had plenty of money and opportunity to conduct pertinent studies, they just haven't been obligated to do so. In regards to government funding, hundreds of millions of dollars have been spent on research into vaccine hesitancy and on advertising campaigns aimed to build trust in the genetic vaccines.[249] Why not address hesitancy by conducting studies that would actually provide a better assessment of the true risk of myocarditis/pericarditis and other serious adverse vaccine effects that have been flagged? Instead, authorities have discounted people's concerns and relied on passive databases that may underestimate rates by a factor of a hundred or more.[250] And when massive signals surfaced in the passive databases, they too were discounted. That's no way to build trust.

The priority hasn't been about safety or efficacy. It has been about getting as many people vaccinated as possible, through whatever means necessary with billions of dollars wasted in that pursuit.

As of May 2022, about half of the estimated $5 billion worth of COVID-19 doses made it into the arms of Canadians, with over a $1 billion worth either already expired or set to expire by the end of 2022, and over a $1 billion more in surplus that Canada hoped to donate to other countries before they too expired.[251] These amounts don't even include doses Canada committed to purchase for delivery up to and including the 2023-24 fiscal year. Moreover, billions of dollars have been put towards the WHO's *Access to COVID-19 Tools Accelerator* and other international vaccine initiatives in support of vaccine procurement, production, delivery and distribution worldwide.[252]

Safeguard Failure #4: Patient-Oriented Medical Care

Physicians were unable to question vaccine safety and efficacy or use their own medical judgment when issuing vaccine exemptions to patients.

Assertions that the new genetic vaccines were "safe and effective" have been, for the most part, hollow and disingenuous.

"Safe and effective" is meaningless without specifying what is meant by those terms. Certainly, the vaccines have been shown not to be effective in reducing transmission and many individuals do not regard the vaccines as safe based on the safety concerns already flagged by Health Canada to date.

Given the huge knowledge gaps with these vaccines, many were left wondering how authorities could proclaim the pharmaceuticals safe and effective. The assurance of product safety has been particularly suspect since: (i) the vaccines were approved with no mid or long-term safety data; (ii) the clinical trials were unblinded after six months; (iii) no active tracking systems had been set up to adequately track and monitor vaccine effects; (iv) passive post-market surveillance systems such as the Vaccine Adverse Event Reporting System (VAERS) in the United States, EudraVigilance in the European Union, and Yellow Card in the United Kingdom had picked up huge safety signals; and (v) Pfizer's own pharmacovigilance documents show that by June 2022, the company was aware of almost 5 million adverse events covering nearly every organ system — about 27% of them serious and debilitating.[253]

These glaring issues didn't stop public health agencies across Canada from asserting that the vaccines were *proven* safe and effective. The provincial colleges that regulate physicians and surgeons across Canada also made that strong claim and expected their members to accept it as gospel.[254] But where's the proof?

On scientific grounds such claims could have been disputed... but not by a physician or surgeon without risk of reprimand or possibly losing their license to practice medicine. Whether a physician assessed the vaccine to be in the best interests of a patient or not, they were not free to use their own medical judgment to grant a COVID-19 vaccine exemption. Only those individuals with narrowly defined medical conditions as stipulated in the college guidelines qualified for an exemption.

Safeguard Failure #5: Research Institutes & Journals

> **Academic honesty and public health were forfeited in lieu of a politicized vaccine agenda.**

In terms of assessing the ability of the new genetic vaccines to curb transmission and to reduce hospitalization and death, the vast majority of studies fail the most basic tests of statistical inference. There's no way around the fact that authorities could not back much of what they were saying from a scientific or evidential standpoint. It has been shocking to witness how far researchers and research institutions were willing to twist and manipulate data to help push a largely unsuccessful product onto people.

A plethora of studies have emerged claiming the vaccines to be a tremendous success. Such studies artificially prop up the "safe and effective" mantra. But the **many critical scientific shortcomings** experienced during the clinical trial phase cannot be overcome with an armory of sub-standard observational studies, model simulations and counterfactual make-believe scenarios.

The performance variables used for most observational studies (i.e. COVID-19 cases, COVID-19 deaths, COVID-19 hospitalizations) are inherently unreliable, easily manipulated and designed to skew public opinion in favour of vaccination. There is an under-appreciation for the huge number of confounding variables at play, an issue that only gets worse over time. Such observational studies provide suggestive evidence at best. At worst they are misleading and contribute to psychological manipulation to convince everyone, regardless of age, health, and need, to take a drug that has not been shown to be in their best interest.

Model simulations and counterfactual models, on the other hand, do not provide evidence of anything at all — they are hypothetical.

There are many ways to conduct a poor study. Pointing to a vast amount of poor-quality, critically flawed research that supports a conjecture does not make the conjecture true. So far, government and public health officials have failed to produce studies that *prove* their claims of safety and efficacy. Many competent scientists are ready and willing to debate the flawed scientific evidence that has been used to peddle the genetic vaccines to the public. However, there appears to be steadfast resistance by pro-mandate institutions and officials to have an open and honest discussion. My attempts and the attempts of many other scientists to engage in such discourse have failed. Institutions and key figureheads have the power to simply shut out opposition, disregard evidence and in many cases earn promotions while the public pays the price.

Fisman's fraudulent transmission study provides a glaring example of the unscientific "evidence" that top academic and medical institutions are willing to accept and promote to fulfill the government's politically-driven vaccine agenda. More importantly, it indicates a severe lack of real evidence to back their position.

While individuals in key positions in society have backed mass COVID-19 vaccination, it should be noted that many researchers and scientists across Canada have voiced scientifically-sound concerns about the new genetic vaccines. Unfortunately, a good many of those who opted to not subject their body to the substance were ostracized, put on unpaid leave or forced out of their jobs altogether — one sure way to achieve scientific "consensus" among those who remain.

Ultimate Safeguard Failure: The Charter & The Courts

The government gamed the system to circumvent Charter protections.

Prior to the pandemic, Canadians were free to choose not to take a pharmaceutical they didn't want. Certainly, if an individual researched a drug and was not satisfied with its safety record or convinced of its usefulness, that person could simply not take it and continue on with daily life without reprimand. As an additional layer of protection, Canada's drug approval process helped safeguard against dangerous pharmaceuticals reaching the market. Healthy individuals were able to enjoy sports, recreation and reap the benefits of living a healthy lifestyle. They weren't considered a disease threat to others and they certainly weren't expected to undergo medical treatments or take drugs in order to participate in normal daily activities.

With the advent of vaccine passports and mandates, all that changed.

First, Health Canada loosened its safety and efficacy requirements to usher in the new genetic vaccines. Then, the government demanded that every Canadian age 12 and older take them in order to live normally. Both the federal and provincial governments were able to circumvent Charter protections that sought to guarantee an individual the right to freely choose *not* to take a drug they didn't want, need, or deem safe. In essence, the government turned from providing a measure of protection against dangerous or unwanted pharmaceuticals to becoming a threat to anyone who refused to take the new COVID-19 drugs.

Under the guise of public good, and after a successful scapegoating campaign, the government essentially took away many individuals' right to say "no" when it came to what went into their own body. To those who suffered the consequences under this new regime, the vaccine mandates and passports felt like a complete subversion of justice where the executive power of government bi-passed courts, virtually convicted the unvaccinated and went straight to sentencing and punishment. Guilty of what? Misogyny, as Trudeau claimed? Acting like reckless, intoxicated, syphilis carrying drivers, as Fisman alluded to? — *It didn't matter. The reasons were fluid and made up as they went along.*

The pandemic has exposed a major gap in the Charter's ability to adequately protect Canadians from government overreach, especially as it pertains to bodily autonomy. The next chapter explores some of the ways the government was able to circumvent Charter protections, discusses how the Fisman study fits into the picture, and highlights the need to reinforce basic rights' protections.

CHAPTER 13

Circumventing Charter Protections

"The judicial branch has, in its finest hours, stood firmly on the side of individuals against those who would trample their rights."

— *Herb Kohl, US Senator & Businessman (1935–)*

Prior to the pandemic, the legal establishment widely held the view that mandatory vaccination was unconstitutional. In the 1996 Canadian National Report on Immunization, lawyers for the Department of Health specifically stated that vaccination "cannot be made mandatory because of the Canadian Constitution."[255] Indeed, as late as May of 2021 Trudeau publicly stated: "We're not a country that makes vaccination mandatory." That same month, Privacy Commissioner Daniel Therrien said compulsory vaccination was "an encroachment on civil liberties" that breaches the Privacy Act.[256] His comments were in line with the basic principle that compulsory disclosure of medical information is a "massive violation of privacy."[257]

Less than six months later the federal government imposed a mandatory COVID-19 vaccination policy for federal employees and banned the unvaccinated from travelling by plane, train or boat. They did so without legal precedent and without a demonstrated need. I, like many other Canadians, was left wondering how that was possible. Why didn't the Charter protect us?

Are the Courts Truly Impartial?

Following the WHO's declaration of a global COVID-19 pandemic, court operations in Canada were significantly curtailed. To reduce the transmission of the novel coronavirus, courts across Canada closed their doors to the public.[258] This included the Federal Court and the Supreme Court of Canada. Most court operations were shut down with hearings limited to the most urgent matters.

About two months later, Canada's top judge, Chief Justice Richard Wagner of the Supreme Court of Canada, paired up with Liberal MP David Lametti, Minister of Justice and Attorney General of Canada, to establish an Action Committee on Court Operations in Response to COVID-19.[259] The committee's main purpose was to help restore the full operation of Canadian courts while ensuring the safety of court users and staff. A central component of the Action Committee mandate read as follows:[260]

The Action Committee will adapt public health principles and guidelines identified by First Ministers and health authorities to the unique context of courts, providing national guidance to support the restoration and stabilization of court operations in all jurisdictions.

The Action Committee was comprised of senior-level judiciary, including chief provincial and federal court judges, alongside senior-level participation by federal and provincial governments. The committee provided provincial, territorial, and judicial decision-makers with health and safety information and court-specific guidelines.

On September 2, 2021, Canada's Federal Court became the first court to publicly disclose the COVID-19 vaccination status of its judges and prothonotaries — all fully vaccinated.[261]

The 53 members of the Federal Court are pleased to inform the public that we are all fully vaccinated against COVID-19.

— *Federal Court of Canada, September 2, 2021*[262]

A few days later, *prior* to the federal vaccine mandate, the Supreme Court of Canada imposed its own COVID-19 vaccination mandate for in-court staff, as directed by Chief Justice Richard Wagner. The top court also announced that all nine of its judges were fully vaccinated.[263]

Under a constitutional challenge, will the courts rule against the very measures that they themselves adopted whole-heartedly? Are the courts truly impartial?

Instead of defaulting to the long held notion that mandatory vaccination was unconstitutional, the Supreme Court of Canada, under the guidance of the federal government, imposed vaccination requirements onto their own staff. While the Action Committee's terms of reference recognized that judicial independence is a fundamental constitutional principle, their actions indicate a worrisome lack of independence. The Action Committee was informed by government representatives, not an independent, objective body. The courts readily adopted controversial policies that millions of citizens across the country have rejected as violating the supreme law of Canada.

Side-stepping the Burden of Proof

Section 1 of the Charter includes a provision of reasonable limits to individual rights and freedoms when it is in the best interest of the greater community. However, that provision puts **the onus of proof on the government** to show that any such limits are "demonstrably justified" via the Oakes test. While some may believe that a declaration by the WHO of a pandemic and global health emergency provides justification for drastic restrictions, on its own it does not. As far as Section 1 of the Charter is concerned, such a declaration is neither necessary nor sufficient, though it no doubt sways public opinion and influences the courts. The question is: Do the restrictions satisfy the criteria as set out in the Oakes test (i.e. are the limitations pressing and necessary, rational, proportionate and not overly broad)?

Despite the burden of proof resting with the government to justify infringements on civil liberties, courts are reluctant to nullify laws that were enacted for the public good.

> *Courts will not lightly order that laws that Parliament or a legislature has duly enacted for the public good are inoperable in advance of complete constitutional review, which is always a complex and difficult matter.*

— *Harper v. Canada (Attorney General), [2000] 2 S.C.R. 764, at para. 9*[264]

Thus, while cases make their way through the courts, challenged laws may continue to play out under the presumption that they support a public good.[265] In this regard, a sluggish legal process helps to prolong potential human rights violations. In cases involving COVID-19 vaccination, some courts have gone even further, aiding questionable government policies by taking judicial notice of the safety, efficacy and overall benefit of the new genetic vaccines.

Judicial notice means accepting a fact without proof. It is supposed to apply to facts that are clearly uncontroversial or beyond reasonable dispute. Certainly, this is not the case when it comes to much of the evidence upon which the government based its vaccine policies, including the safety and efficacy of the rushed-to-market COVID-19 vaccines. Taking judicial notice of unproven notions that are central to the issue under dispute is extremely prejudicial. Facts judicially noticed are not proved by evidence under oath; nor are they tested by cross-examination (R. v. J.M., 2021).[266] This is at odds with Section 1 that puts the burden of proof onto the government.

Superior Court Justice J. Christopher Corkery expressed serious concerns about the court taking judicial notice of government information. In doing so, he provided numerous examples of erroneous and harmful state actions that dispel the notion that our government is always right, including:[267]

- The residential school system where Indigenous children were taken away from their families while government and much of society chose to stay wilfully blind to the abuse the children suffered for decades — "We're still finding children's bodies."

- Sterilizing Inuit women.

- Canada's approval of the "perfectly safe" experimental drug thalidomide in the late 1950's that caused thousands of birth defects and dead babies before it was withdrawn from the market.

- Japanese and Chinese internment camps during World War II.

Interment camps — is that where Canada was headed with the unvaccinated? For many of us, it sure felt that way.

> *"Emergencies can be used by governments to justify a lot of things that later turn out to be wrong."*
> *— Justice J.C. Corkery, August 5, 2022*

Justice Corkery's open acknowledgment of our government's history of human rights atrocities provided a much needed reminder that the government and its experts are far from infallible and that one of the courts' primary duties is to catch and correct their mistakes.

> *The list of grievous government mistakes and miscalculations is both endless and notorious. Catching and correcting those mistakes is one of the most important functions of an independent judiciary.*
>
> *— M.M. v. W.A.K., 2022 ONSC 4580, para 39*

Justice Corkery made the cautionary remarks while presiding over a case involving a mother and father who were at odds regarding the COVID-19 vaccination of their 12 year old daughter who did not wish to receive the injection. The father sought a court order that would direct the mother to ensure that their daughter got vaccinated as per the government's recommendations. Unlike many other courts where rulings had relied on taking judicial notice of the safety and efficacy of COVID-19 vaccines, Justice Corkery was not prepared to simply take the government at its word. "How can you take judicial notice of a moving target?" he aptly stated. Without the prejudicial declaration, the judge found no evidence to support the notion that it was in the child's best interest that she receive the vaccine.

Government experts sound so sure of themselves in recommending the current vaccines. But they were equally sure when they told us to line up for AstraZeneca. Now they don't even mention that word.

— Court Justice J. Christopher Corkery (M.M. v. W.A.K., 2022)

Unfortunately, the impartiality exhibited by Justice Corkery has been a rare trait amongst justices presiding over challenges involving pandemic measures; equally rare is his healthy skepticism of recommendations put forth by government experts.

"Public Good": Unproven. Untested. Unquantified.

"Public good" — an overly broad, unspecified concept that has been used by politicians to give blanket justification for all pandemic restrictions. While such claims are to be expected by politicians, the presumption of "public good" by the courts is *highly* problematic.

Since most people were not at serious risk from the virus, the government's COVID-19 vaccine drive was dependent on fostering a sense of collective benefit to justify infringements on individual rights. But public benefit was never established nor quantified for the vaccine mandates or passports, though the notion has been ingrained into the public psyche through endless repetition in the media.

Initially, the public good argument for COVID-19 vaccination hinged on the vaccines' ability to curb transmission. Once that primary benefit became highly questionable, authorities emphasized indirect, second-order benefits stemming from the vaccines' purported ability to reduce illness and death. Theoretically, these reductions might lead to fewer hospitalizations, thus reducing the burden on the health care system, and could lead to a reduction in employee absenteeism, thus safeguarding service levels in key sectors such as health care and transportation.

As discussed in Chapter 5, the vaccines' ability to reduce illness and death were never scientifically established, and there is significant evidence to the contrary. But, even had these benefits been proven, such gains wouldn't necessarily translate into material impacts on health care and service delivery. Moreover, when leveraging these presumed benefits to justify vaccine mandates and restrictions, the state would need to go a step further and show that the measures imposed would enhance such benefits enough to justify infringements on individual rights. Since it is mainly the elderly and those with comorbid conditions that are at risk of serious complications from COVID-19, establishing such indirect second and third-order benefits for working-aged adults would be exceedingly difficult. That is, even had the vaccines been fully effective in preventing serious illness and death, the state would've had a very difficult time demonstrating that workplace <u>mandates</u> — not just the vaccines — were sufficiently targeted to make a difference in the vulnerable population and that they would lead to a meaningful increase in the public benefits claimed. The same is true for any restriction placed on the general public.

Furthermore, if federal, provincial and municipal governments were able to overcome this huge hurdle, they would still need to demonstrate that their mandates or restrictions weren't arbitrary. The reality is, many factors contribute to one's overall health and impact the likelihood of needing medical care or taking time off work, such as: exercise, eating habits, alcohol consumption etc. Yet, the government doesn't impose mandates on those personal health choices. Simply stated, relying on these second and third-order public benefits to justify mandates invites a tidal wave of counter-arguments and is fraught with logical and legal inconsistencies.

> *Without a demonstrated reduction in transmission, the benefits shift from communal to personal and, as such, individual rights become paramount.*

The unearned presumption of public benefit naturally confers a sense that the vaccines are "safe and effective" and that upholding the policy or policies in question is the more cautious approach. That some courts have gone so far as to take judicial notice of the safety and effectiveness is a stunning move given the controversial evidence. If it is assumed the policies are in the best interests of the public and that the vaccines are safe and effective, then the potential harms stemming from vaccine policies may not be fully considered or appreciated. The far-reaching possibility that the policies may actually be detrimental to society as a whole escapes consideration.

The presumption of public good is pervasive and highly prejudicial in any litigation in which Charter rights are a central issue.

It is important to realize that the presumption of public good is pervasive — it comes into play both directly as well as indirectly through reliance on previous court rulings grounded on the presumption. That is, bias is pushed forward to future cases, thus compounding the prejudice.

The purpose of the Charter is to protect the rights and freedoms of Canadians from government abuse and overreach. In cases challenging the government on Charter violations the presumption of public good is *highly* prejudicial. Indeed, when coupled with a perceived "emergency" situation, it imparts an innate sense that highly restrictive policies are reasonably justified. That perception puts a greater burden on the individual whose rights have been infringed upon to prove that such policies resulted in an overreach of power. This shifting of the onus of proof from the government onto the individual is contrary to Section 1 of the Charter.[268]

The presumption of public good leads to situations in which rights and freedoms may be violated for years until a complete constitutional review is undertaken, if one gets undertaken at all. In the case of travel restrictions, we've witnessed how this apparent incongruence can be exploited by the government.

Did Government Game the System?

Before Section 1 of the Charter is engaged a finding must first be made that a right or freedom has been limited. Prior to COVID-19 it was a given that mandatory vaccination was unconstitutional under Section 7 of the Charter, which protects an individual's right to life, liberty and security of the person:

Section 7: Everyone has the right to life, liberty and security of the person and the right not to be deprived thereof except in accordance with the principles of fundamental justice.

The right to life is engaged whenever state action imposes increased risk of death, either directly or indirectly. *The right to liberty* includes the right to make reasonable medical choices without fear of government reprisal. *Security of the person* includes a person's right to control their own bodily integrity, both physical and psychological. It is engaged when the state imposes an unwanted medical treatment or fundamentally deprives a person of the ability to earn a livelihood.[269]

In October 2021, the Government of Canada imposed a COVID-19 vaccination requirement for federal public servants. As stated on the official government website, the objectives of the mandate were to:[270]

1. Take every precaution reasonable, in the circumstances, for the protection of the health and safety of employees. Vaccination is a key element in the protection of employees against COVID-19;

2. Improve the vaccination rate across Canada of employees in the core public administration through COVID-19 vaccination; and

3. Given that operational requirements may include ad hoc onsite presence, all employees, including those working remotely and teleworking must be fully vaccinated to protect themselves, colleagues, and clients from COVID-19 (with exceptions based on medical or prohibited grounds for discrimination).

Basically, the objectives of the federal vaccine mandate were to: increase vaccination of employees, and, to protect employees and clients from COVID-19 through vaccination.

The mandate applied to the Core Public Administration, including members of the Royal Canadian Mounted Police. It also applied to employees in federally regulated transport industries. Other federally regulated workplaces, the Canadian Armed Forces, Crown corporations and separate agencies were being directed by the Trudeau government to implement vaccine policies mirroring the requirements.[271]

What About the Principles of Fundamental Justice?

Any restriction in the inalienable rights protected under Section 7 must be in accordance with fundamental principles of justice, which concern: arbitrariness, overbreadth and gross disproportionality. On its face, all three objectives stipulated by the government's vaccine mandate appear incompatible with that requirement.

Was mandating vaccination reasonable under the circumstances?

By fall of 2021, the infection fatality rate of COVID-19 was estimated to be about 0.05% for individuals under 70 yrs,[272] in line with influenza. The median age of a "COVID-19 death" was above 80 yrs, and over 90% of deaths occurred in individuals with one or more comorbid conditions.[273] These statistics indicate that, not only were workplace mandates unnecessary, but only an infinitesimal benefit was even possible for those in the workforce. Meanwhile, mounting concerns and profuse uncertainties in the health risks associated with the new genetic vaccines surfaced, adding to the unease regarding the complete lack of long-term safety data.

In short, most working-aged individuals were at fairly low risk of serious complications from the actual virus and the COVID-19 vaccines were known to produce a range of adverse reactions, some severe, including death.[274] Can it truly be considered reasonable to mandate a new genetic vaccine for such a poor trade off? —*No.*

The infection fatality rate for COVID-19 was comparable to the seasonal flu. Such a mandate had never been imposed in the federal sector for the flu vaccine or any other, let alone an experimental one. The COVID-19 mandate was overbreadth; the penalties, including unpaid leave and invasion of privacy rights, grossly disproportionate.

Was mandatory COVID-19 vaccination rationally connected to the stated objective of increased health, safety and protection of employees?

As discussed throughout this book, there was no solid evidence to support the assertion that vaccination leads to reduced community transmission. Without that link, the argument cannot be made that mandatory vaccination would help protect coworkers or provide increased safety in the work environment. At the time of implementation, the mandate was irrational and thus arbitrary. Moreover, there was evidence it may, in fact, be counterproductive.

Real-world data at the time the policy was implemented indicated that any immunity imparted by the vaccines waned after about six months, that a vaccinated individual could still get sick and still be contagious, and that fully vaccinated individuals may be as transmissive as unvaccinated individuals. In fact, there were already indications out of the UK that, under certain conditions, transmission may even be greater amongst the vaccinated.[275]

It is worth noting that the majority of Canadians received their second dose in June and July of 2021 which would, according to the waning statistics, make them susceptible to COVID-19 by Dec 2021—Jan 2022, just in time for the flu season. Indeed, Canada went on to witness a drastic surge in cases during that exact period with the Omicron variant.

Is improving the vaccination rate an important or necessary goal in and of itself?

Objective 2, to improve the vaccination rate through COVID-19 vaccination, can be rephrased as follows: (1) to increase drug uptake by mandating the drug, or, (2) to increase the uptake of a medical treatment by mandating the treatment, or, (3) to increase the vaccination rate by depriving employees the option not to vaccinate (technically the unvaccinated would still be called "employees", they just wouldn't be on the payroll).

Vaccination for the sake of vaccination, without being tied to a health or safety objective, in and of itself does not constitute an important or necessary goal. Mandating a vaccine for the sole purpose of achieving greater vaccination is simply the state vetoing the inalienable right to bodily autonomy.

Was mandating vaccines for those working remotely or teleworking rational?

Mandating a vaccine to those working remotely or teleworking would be extremely hard to justify under any circumstance. Certainly, if a person works remotely and never physically interacts with coworkers, there is no possibility of transmitting any virus to them. For those who may have had to interact with coworkers or clients on occasion, less invasive measures such as rapid antigen testing were available.

Not only were those working remotely not exempt from the mandate, but those who had acquired natural immunity were not exempt either, which made no rational sense whatsoever. It is worth noting that if the policy is shown to be overbreadth or grossly disproportionate for a single person then it violates Section 7 (Bedford, 2013, para 111, 113, 121, 122).

On their surface, the federal objectives themselves were ill-conceived and appear to breach Section 7 of the Charter. A deeper dive into the policy reveals many other logical inconsistencies, too many to cover here.

It is important to bear in mind that Section 7 was designed to protect individual interests. Societal interests or matters of public policy such as health care costs and service levels should be considered under Section 1 not Section 7 (Government of Canada as cited in R. v. Malmo-Levine, R. v. Caine, [2003] at paragraph 98;[276] Canada v. Bedford. [2013] 125-126).[277]

Prior to the pandemic, there had been no Supreme Court of Canada decisions that directly upheld a Section 7 violation under Section 1 of the Charter.[278]

The rights protected by Section 7 are "basic to our conception of a free and democratic society, and hence are not easily overridden by competing social interests." (Charkaoui v. Canada, 2007)[279]

Re-defining Charter Rights & The Law

One argument that has been used by those imposing vaccine mandates is that there was no Section 7 violation because the employee (or student in the case of university mandates) was not forced to take the injection. They assert that people had a choice of whether or not to vaccinate, even if that choice was between two undesirable outcomes.

Consider the words of Prime Minister Trudeau following the suspension of the federal COVID-19 vaccine mandates:

> *And therefore, while not forcing anyone to get vaccinated, I chose to make sure that all the incentives and all of the protections were there to encourage Canadians to get vaccinated. And that's exactly what they did.*

> — *Trudeau, April 2023*[280]

Trudeau claimed that he didn't "force" anyone to get vaccinated. Many disagree. While he may not have physically held people down and injected them with a vaccine, that is not a requirement for a Section 7 violation. Not only is the right to life protected under Section 7, so too is bodily integrity and the right to make reasonable medical choices free of reprisal. Did the mandates coerce or cause some individuals to do something against their will? —*Certainly.*

It is important to assess what options were available to the individual at the time in order to determine whether or not a meaningful choice actually existed.

> *The most important factors in determining the procedural content of fundamental justice in a given case are the nature of the legal rights at issue and the severity of the consequences to the individuals concerned.*

> — *Singh v. Minister of Employment & Immigration, 1985*[281]

Trudeau's repeated claims that people had a choice is of little value when that choice was not a meaningful one. Box 6 presents a summary of Trudeau's "incentive" program for COVID-19 vaccination of federal employees. It is important to note that the onus is on governments to select

Box 6: Federal Vaccine Mandate
Meaningful Choice or Extortion?

The federal government is Canada's single largest employer.

In the fall of 2021, the federal government mandated the COVID-19 vaccination of all federal public servants and employees in federally regulated transport industries.

Mandatory vaccination applied whether employees were teleworking, working remotely or working on-site.

Crown corporations and other employers in the federally regulated sector were instructed to implement vaccination policies for their employees that mirrored requirements for the Core Public Admin.

Together, an estimated 19,000 employers and 1,235,000 employees were subject to COVID-19 vaccination policies.[282] Non-compliant employees were to be placed on **leave without pay.**

The federal government **disqualified unvaccinated persons from accessing employment insurance benefits.**

The federal government banned unvaccinated persons age 12 and older from travelling by plane or train in Canada.

The federal government offered provinces $1 billion to implement vaccine passport systems restricting unvaccinated persons from social venues, sport and recreational facilities etc.

Other employers, such as some hospitals and universities, also mandated the COVID-19 vaccination for their employees.

In many industries, COVID-19 vaccination was required for new hires.

From February 2020 to July 2022, 86.7% of all new jobs were in the public sector with almost no net job creation in the private sector,[283] thus severely limiting job prospects for the unvaccinated.

the least harmful or restrictive measures that can reasonably be expected to achieve the desired outcome.

Reframing punishments and irrational consequences as incentives and encouragement does not change the punitive nature of the federal vaccine mandate. On multiple occasions, Trudeau publicly threatened federal employees with punishment, including placing them on unpaid leave, if they tried to exercise their right to bodily autonomy and chose to forgo COVID-19 vaccination.[284] Once re-elected, he followed through with those threats, as well as numerous other ultimatums. Trudeau's actions demonstrate that the federal government did not view vaccination as an individual right that is protected from reprisal.

Not only did the federal vaccine mandate appear to violate Section 7, but it did so many times over — a cascade of compound violations. Unreasonable medical coercion and infringement on one's right to medical privacy (covered under Sections 7 & 8) were just the tip of the iceberg.

Given the largely incomplete safety profile of the vaccines and the inadequate information regarding their health risks, there is doubt whether a recipient could truly provide informed consent. Moreover, consent must be voluntary, free of any suggestion of duress or coercion[285] — yet another violation.

Not only did the Trudeau government cut off the employment income of non-compliant employees, they encouraged other employers to do the same to their unvaccinated workers. Then, to top off the financial assault, the feds went out of their way to ensure the "anti-vaxxers" were denied employment insurance benefits.[286] Given the state of the economy at the time, especially for the unvaccinated, such drastic penalties may be seen as depriving individuals of "economic rights fundamental to human survival"[287] — yet another violation of Section 7.

How does unimaginable stress and the prospect of financial ruin protect the health and safety of employees?

The psychological dimension of Section 7 should not be overlooked. There's no doubt the vaccine mandates caused extreme stress and anxiety for many federal workers, not only due to the financial penalties that were imposed, but by the deep sense of betrayal and the demeaning way they were treated. For many, the implementation of the mandates effectively made known their vaccination status to coworkers, and the prime minister's very public condemnation of the unvaccinated all but ensured such individuals would be stigmatized — psychological integrity is covered under Section 7, security of the person.

The vaccine mandates together with vaccine passports created an identifiable group, the unvaccinated, who endured immense discrimination — a seeming violation of Section 15.

Some individuals asked for an exemption to the vaccine mandate based on religious or conscientious grounds and were denied — a possible violation of Section 2a, the right to freedom of conscience or religion.

The added travel restrictions against the unvaccinated brings in violations under Section 6 — mobility rights.

These violations are in addition to the restrictions endured over the pre-mandate phase of the pandemic (lockdowns, school closures, capacity limits within one's own household etc).

For many Canadians, the government's actions during the pandemic felt like an unbridled assault on their fundamental human rights and freedoms. The Charter proved to be of little value.

It is worth noting that the federal government's "incentive" of placing employees on leave without pay while simultaneously denying them employment insurance benefits is not only subject to Charter considerations but also employment law. Most employers do not have the right to suspend their employees from work unless it's explicitly detailed in their employee's contract. Moreover, suspensions must be reasonable and justified with the burden of proof to demonstrate this resting with the employer.[288] Unfortunately, many employers paid no heed to that requirement.

Keeping Challenges Out of the Courts

In cases pertaining to vaccine mandates in the workplace, many factors weigh into decisions involving infringements on civil liberties. How challenges to such policies are handled greatly depends on whether the workers challenging them are unionized or not.

The public sector and federally regulated industries are highly unionized in Canada. This has allowed challenges to COVID-19 vaccine mandates brought forward by unions or unionized workers to stay out of the courts. Unionized workers are instructed to go through their union's grievance process. Unions, in turn, are to go through administrative tribunals instead of the courts. Such cases are decided by labour arbitrators. Courts intervene only when there is a gap in the legislative regime, i.e., when an adequate alternative remedy is unavailable through the appropriate administrative tribunal.[289] Several court applications involving mandatory COVID-19 vaccination have been dismissed on the grounds that courts lack the necessary jurisdiction.

Unfortunately, the presumption of "public good" and acceptance of the fictitious conjecture that vaccine mandates reduce the spread of COVID-19 have often factored into the decision-making process with arbitrators erring on the side of employers.[290] Worse, there have been several arbitrations or tribunals in which unions supposedly representing unvaccinated members did not challenge the easily refutable expert evidence presented by the employers (Toronto Professional Fire Fighters' Association, I.A.A.F. Local 3888 and City of Toronto, 2022;[291] City of Toronto and Toronto Civic Employees' Union, CUPE, Local 416;[292] and, United Steelworkers Local 2008 v. Attorney General of Canada, 2022,[293] to name a few).

If unions aren't going to challenge the employer's expert evidence regarding safety, efficacy and necessity of the vaccines, then why bother challenging the mandates at all?

The evident failure of the vaccines to curb the spread of the Omicron variant hasn't escaped notice of all arbitrators, however. In FCA Canada Inc. v Unifor (2022), the arbitrator ruled that the two-dose vaccine requirement was unreasonable since it was no longer effective against transmission.[294]

More recently, a military tribunal found the Canadian Armed Forces' COVID-19 vaccine mandate violated the Charter rights of members who refused vaccination, ruling the policy to be "arbitrary" and "overly broad."[295] The tribunal also determined that the limitations were not justified under Section 1. Though significant, the tribunal's findings are non-binding; the final decision lies with the Chief of the Defence Staff.[296]

While the ruling in the military tribunal is encouraging, many Canadians find it disheartening that the government has been able to exploit the perceived pandemic emergency, jurisdiction limits, and the sluggish court system to impose such detrimental measures. Even more concerning, the inappropriate presumption of public good and judicial notice regarding safety and efficacy of the vaccines have greatly alleviated the government's burden of proof in establishing whether their highly restrictive measures were necessary, rational, proportionate and not overly broad (as per Oakes test).

Gaming the System

A court review of the government's decision to impose a travel ban against unvaccinated Canadians had been scheduled for the fall of 2022. For the millions of Canadians affected, that would've marked the first time the government would be made to present its case for one of the country's most discriminatory policies against the unvaccinated.

Four separate court challenges had been filed against Transport Canada's civil aviation travel restrictions; the Federal Court of Canada was set to hear them all at the same time. The mandate factum put together by the four parties along with the testimony of government experts during the discovery process highlighted the exceedingly flimsy evidential basis for the restrictions.[297] The government's own experts admitted that the restrictions allowed COVID-19 infected vaccinated people on airplanes while uninfected unvaccinated individuals were prohibited. Moreover, the documents indicate that the Public Health Agency of Canada never recommended the vaccine mandate to Transport Canada. Those in the transport sector who worked on the construction of the interim orders admitted to being unaware of any actual evidence to support the vaccine requirement that would severely restrict the mobility rights of millions of Canadians. With such admissions, one is left to wonder if it ever occurred to the government that they may one day have to defend their position.

The cross-examinations of government witnesses were quite revealing. Jennifer Little, the director general of COVID Recovery at Transport Canada, was responsible for crafting the policy that she called "one of the strongest vaccination mandates for travellers in the world." Ms. Little was not at liberty to say who had given her team the order to impose the travel mandate, citing "cabinet confidence."[298] The lack of scientific justification for the travel restrictions along with the suggestion that a senior official in the prime minister's cabinet had ordered the Transport Canada team to impose the mandate indicates a purely political play.

In mid-June 2022, just as the cross-examinations of government witnesses were wrapping up, the Government of Canada announced the suspension of the vaccination requirements for domestic and outbound travel. Within days of the suspension, government lawyers filed a motion seeking to shut down the court challenge on the grounds that it was now moot. They succeeded. Associate Chief Justice Jocelyne Gagne ruled in their favour in late October 2022, just days before the constitutional challenge was to begin.[299] The voices of the wronged would not be heard — outweighed by the expenditure that a five-day hearing would incur.[300] An appeal has been scheduled for October 2023.

This is a monumental case for Canadian democracy. If the appeal is successful, the government will finally be required to prove their restrictions were necessary and reasonable — a hugely difficult task in light of all the evidence to the contrary.

If the appeal fails, then the Federal Court of Canada would be allowing the government to get away with gaming the system. It would effectively legitimize the practice of restricting constitutionally protected rights so long as the restrictions are removed before the courts, moving at a snail's pace, have a chance to hold the government accountable. It gets worse. The government made it clear the restrictions were merely suspended and that they can be reinstated at any time if they believe the circumstances warrant them.

Impose restrictions on civil rights and liberties. Claim it's for the public good. Suspend restrictions on the eve of the court challenge. Have the court declare the case moot. Rinse. Repeat. … until the right can be taken away altogether.

When Rights Become Privileges

During a campaign stop in August 2021, Trudeau made specific reference to the privileges that would be given to those granted vaccine passports funded by his government. It was an interesting word choice — referring to civil liberties as privileges — coming from a man who has claimed to choose his words carefully.

> *The Federal Government has announced that we're gonna pay for the development of those privileges that you get once you get vaccinated because everyone needs to get vaccinated & those (unvaccinated) people are putting us all at risk.*
>
> — *Justin Trudeau, campaigning 2021*[301]

Throughout the pandemic, the government did indeed treat Charter rights and freedoms as privileges to be granted to Canadians conditionally as opposed to fundamental pillars of our society that are to be protected from reprisal. This **authoritarian** shift away from core democratic values was particularly jarring with the introduction of vaccine mandates. As noted by the United Nations General Assembly, not only is bodily autonomy a human right, it is the foundation upon which other human rights are built (as witnessed by the cascading violations that occurred when it wasn't respected). Moreover, respect for autonomy is a core tenet of international medical ethics.[302]

Apparently, the provincial and federal governments didn't see it that way, at least not in regard to vaccination.

If vaccine choice were no longer regarded as an individual right in Canada, then vaccine mandates would not violate Charter rights and there would be no onus on the government to justify their use via Oakes test. Moreover, there would be little standing in the way of general population mandates. That is, instead of being presented little choice, Canadians could be provided with no choice at all.

That certainly appeared to be the direction Canada was heading. The federal government was gearing up for such talks to take place with the provinces and territories before the Freedom Convoy rolled into Ottawa.[303] At that time, Federal Health Minister Jean-Yves Duclos was asserting that mandatory vaccine laws could eventually exist in Canada. Meanwhile, on the science front, Fisman's faux study was underway in its attempt to give scientific legitimacy to the notion that vaccine choice should not be considered an individual right and that vaccine mandates were a reasonable and utilitarian undertaking.

.

Fisman's Fraud: Undermining Bodily Autonomy

As Fisman, Tuite and Amoako pointed out in their problematic CMAJ publication, the decision not to receive vaccination is often framed in terms of the rights of individuals to opt out. Indeed, constitutional challenges against vaccine-related restrictions hinge on the core principle that vaccine choice is an individual right.

In discussing the idea behind his team's study, Fisman explained that they thought the "rights" of vaccinated people to be protected from unvaccinated people was missing from the conversation regarding vaccine passports and vaccine mandates.[304] Fisman went on to state that "vaccinated individuals have a right not to have their efforts to protect themselves undermined."[305] But no such right exists in the Charter. There is no fundamental right to have one's efforts protected.

Having bodily autonomy does not mean any person gets to undermine the health, rights or autonomy of others. Each individual is free to accept the COVID-19 vaccine, but they have no right to make that choice for others. Indeed, the myths that bodily autonomy undermines group decision-making and that one person's bodily autonomy could undermine the autonomy of others have been addressed and debunked by the United Nations Population Fund (UNFPA, 2021). In the past, these misconceptions have been used to marginalize communities and deny women, persons with disabilities and ethnic minorities around the world their sexual and reproductive rights. The same principles apply to mandatory vaccination and any other measure that undermines the universal value of bodily autonomy. As pointed out by the UNFPA:

Group decisions cannot circumscribe the rights of individuals, and communities must come together to dismantle laws and practices that deprive individuals of autonomy.

Fisman's paper advocates for the very opposite, relying on fraudulent claims to make that point.

In an attempt to demonstrate that an individual's choice not to take the COVID-19 vaccine undermines the choice others made to take the injection, Fisman and his colleagues concocted a hypothetical scenario where the unvaccinated act as the main transmission vectors, placing the entire community at greater risk of infection. Under this purely contrived situation, the authors assert that even if only a small percentage of the population were to remain unvaccinated, it could lead to a large community outbreak. The unvaccinated would be the dominant source of COVID-19 infections for themselves as well as the vaccinated, no matter how minimal the interaction between the two groups.

The authors further argued that high vaccination rates are even more necessary when vaccines confer imperfect immunity, as in the case with the COVID-19 vaccines. Since vaccinated individuals can still get infected so long as the virus is in circulation, the researchers contend that strong public policy to enhance vaccine uptake is warranted. It's simply not enough to separate the unvaccinated from the vaccinated, the choice needs to be taken away from the individual completely:

> *The fact that this excess contribution to risk **cannot be mitigated by separating groups** undermines the assertion that vaccine choice is best left to the individual.*
>
> — *Fisman, Tuite & Amoako, CMAJ April 2022*

At the time of Fisman et al.'s preprint, vaccine passports were in full-force, unvaccinated were barred from most indoor public venues and many employers had imposed a vaccine requirement on their workers. It appears that the researchers were advocating for the next phase: mandatory vaccination for the general population for the public good. Based on their demonstration, the researchers concluded that since one's vaccination status impacts the community as a whole, vaccine choice should not be considered an individual right. It was a very simple line of reasoning, void of any nuance or consideration of the harms, benefits and risks of granting the government that kind of control.

The study's foregone conclusion was made possible by limiting the choice of model parameters to values that would produce the desired results, as opposed to examining the full spectrum of possibilities. In doing so, they excluded scenarios more reflective of the reality on the ground. Had they approached their study objectively, it would have shown that vaccination could very well have the opposite effect intended, that there was a possibility of increasing transmission through vaccination. Indeed, that was the very situation playing out in the real-world during the Omicron wave. It would appear, based on the researchers' own logic, that the government's push to have everyone vaccinated had put the community at greater risk of infection thus demonstrating one of the dangers of taking away the right of the individual in choosing a medical procedure and giving it to the state.

Rather ironically, Fisman's study epitomizes exactly why bodily autonomy must be protected.

The Omicron wave demonstrated that Public Health got it wrong when they promised reduced transmission. That politicians got it wrong when they introduced vaccine passports and mandates. That courts got it wrong when they presumed these highly restrictive policies carried a net public benefit.

Fisman's fraudulent study demonstrates just how far pro-vaccine extremists are willing to go to push their anti-rights ideology onto the community.

The resistance of the establishment to come clean with the fraud and set the record straight, along with their continued denial of reality, indicates this assault on an individual's freedom to choose what goes into their own body goes far beyond rogue scientists that have lost their way.

When researchers commit fraud and tell you their "scientific findings" undermine a Charter right, it would be wise to take notice.

Even when endorsed by a leading research institute.

Especially when done during a period of emergency.

Especially when a top medical journal partakes in the deception.

Especially when a public institute funded the study and continues to support the faux findings and its researchers.

What happens when the state takes away individual choice and they get it wrong? The new genetic vaccines were fraught with uncertainties. Yet, state actors made claims of safety and efficacy with arrogant certainty and saw fit to veto the most valued human right in the Charter, the right to life, liberty and security of person.

They were wrong and we paid the price. With our health. With our freedoms. With our lifestyles. With our relationships.

We need added protections to ensure that such transgressions cannot be repeated.

CHAPTER 14

The Takeaway

"Deception is a sort of seduction. In love and war, adultery and espionage, deceit can only succeed if the deceived party is willing, in some way, to be deceived."
— Ben Macintyre, Operation Mincemeat (2010)[306]

The study by David Fisman, Afia Amoako, and Ashleigh Tuite, serves as a prime example of the danger of mixing toxic political ideology with science — the result: unequivocal hate science.

David Fisman, Afia Amoako and Ashleigh R. Tuite concocted a faux scientific model to fabricate data that showed the unvaccinated constitute a disproportionate risk to society, a trend contrary to reality, then proceeded to state the fabricated results as fact in order to inform government policy that defrauds millions of Canadians of basic rights and freedoms.

In essence, the researchers attempted to overwrite the Omicron wave with a fake simulation that showed the opposite trend, one that better aligned with the political narrative that unvaccinated individuals are drivers of transmission, that they constitute a health risk and should be met with punitive restrictions. The researchers leveraged their fraudulent findings and connections to: (1) defame the unvaccinated, (2) undermine the conviction that vaccination is an individual right, and (3) advocate for federal vaccine mandates and travel restrictions as well as the use of vaccine passports.

The main study sparked a media blitz within mere hours of its publication. National and international headlines warned vaccinated people of the risk of mingling with the unvaccinated. The study and media frenzy revived the faux political narrative that the unvaccinated were to blame for the lion's share of COVID-19 infections and transmissions, when in fact fully vaccinated travellers were spreading it around the globe. The false accusations along with the researchers' derogatory comments and comparisons reinforced fear, anger and contempt towards those who chose to forgo the genetic injections. The fraudulent study was cited in Parliament as justification for the extension of the federal travel restrictions against unvaccinated Canadians.

The myth that unvaccinated people pose greater risk to the public is still believed by many and continues to influence policy. While vaccine mandates and travel restrictions were suspended in June 2022, the Government of Canada has warned that such restrictions could be reinstated in the future. In the spring of 2022 provinces dropped their vaccine passports; however, businesses and other organizations could opt to continue requiring proof of vaccination for employment or to receive services. Some chose to prolong the discrimination.

Protections are Needed

Fisman's study embodies many common elements that have been used to inform or justify the government's pandemic response, including: bias, faulty research, unscientific claims, scapegoating and outright fraud. While there has been no shortage of poor quality studies over the course of the pandemic, the Fisman debacle signifies malignant intent behind the faux transmission narrative. Alarmingly, three top institutions spanning academia, medicine, and health research, staunchly supported the overt fraud. They continued to do so in full knowledge that the fabricated results were used to stigmatize and discriminate against an identifiable group with a view to violate basic rights and freedoms. Law enforcement have been reluctant to get involved and courts have allowed the judicial system to be gamed.

Fisman, Tuite and Amoako attempted to use hate science to take away our right to bodily autonomy. The government-funded fraud should trigger action to protect that right.

There is ample evidence to obliviate the claim that COVID-19 vaccines have reduced community transmission, but that is outside the central point. Regardless of one's view on COVID-19 vaccination or what any other research study shows, there is simply no justification for researchers to fabricate results and attempt to pass them off as facts. This act of deceit cannot be defended. The fact that the researchers attempted to use their contrived results to target a vulnerable group for punishment is beyond the pale. That influential institutions would support the fraud, and media would seek to amplify it, indicates the need for strong corrective measures and protections.

The government was able to demand that all Canadians of age twelve and older take an experimental injection to partake in society. From the very start of the pandemic, COVID-19 was known to be a disease that mostly affected the very elderly and those with underlying health conditions. By May of 2020, the CDC had estimated the survival rate to be around 99.7%.[307] For those under the age 70, estimates were in the range of 99.95% (Ioannidis, 2020).[308] If the government can mandate a vaccine against a disease with such a high rate of survival, one that poses little threat to the vast majority of individuals, they can do so for any drug — unless protections are emplaced.

An Eye to the Future

David Fisman, the main researcher and author of the study, has ties to several pharmaceutical companies that stood to benefit from his fraudulent claims and mandatory vaccination stance, including: Seqirus, Pfizer, AstraZeneca and Sanofi-Pasteur. He has also worked with unions and associations seeking special COVID-19 related accommodations and mandatory vaccination policies. Fisman has been recognized as a leader in shaping Canada's pandemic response with active involvement at all levels of government — municipal, provincial and federal.

Going forward, David Fisman has been chosen to lead the Centre for

Pandemic Readiness, one of the three research centers in the newly created Institute for Pandemics. In this role, he will oversee the modelling and forecasting that advises on future pandemics and outbreaks throughout the world. Dr. Ashleigh Tuite will be contributing her expertise to this new enterprise as well.

The degree to which this cancer spreads and takes root depends on the actions taken now. Authorities tasked with taking action against the fraud and misconduct have instead opted to participate in the delusion. The government, in turn, asked the public to trust these experts without question. Will Canadians tolerate the deception?

"Responsibility to yourself means refusing to let others do your thinking, talking, and naming for you; it means learning to respect and use your own brains and instincts; hence, grappling with hard work."
—Adrienne Rich, Poet, essayist & feminist (1929 -2012)

AFTERWORD

Beyond Fisman: The Human Factor

When I began writing this book I had planned to include a discussion on the social impact of the faux pandemic science and anti-freedom movement of which Fisman and his colleagues have played a significant role. That venture quickly became unwieldy.

Far too many people's lives have been turned upside down by the onslaught of scientifically unsupported pandemic measures (attacks) that threatened every aspect of daily life in Canada.

In early 2022, the unrelenting government overreach sparked a nation-wide freedom movement. This grass-roots movement, the Freedom Convoy, exposed the heavy-handed lengths the Trudeau government was willing to go to in order to quash those who challenged their pandemic narrative. The Canadian government's enactment of the Emergency Act (EA) turned a powerful piece of legislation, meant for times of war or national emergency, against peaceful protesters. While the EA proved to be a drastic measure, unfortunately it is indicative of how the entire pandemic response has been managed.

Key to the government's overreach has been the bastardization of science as a means to subvert the Charter and facilitate the conversion of rights into privileges. Sadly, the fraudulent study by Fisman, Tuite and Amoako scrutinized in this book is indicative of the deceptive science that has plagued our nation throughout the pandemic. A particularly effective tactic has been to drown society in a deluge of garbage studies while censoring rational counter voices and cancelling individuals who refuse to play along.

A focused examination of scientific evidence as it pertains to the extreme infringements on Charter rights and freedoms imposed during the pandemic is needed.

We're at a Tipping Point

With COVID-19 measures paused, there is an illusion that such extreme policies and regulations may be a thing of the past — artifacts of a highly exceptional circumstance, a global pandemic, that is now over. Such naive and wishful thinking runs the risk of not taking proper precautions against recurrence.

When pondering whether draconian policies are likely to resurface it is instructive to question: Why wouldn't they?

The government was hugely rewarded during the pandemic, granting itself immense power and control while spending what seemed like endless amounts of money. So far, there has been little (if any) accountability for policy failures and drastic human rights violations. Far from admitting mistakes or any wrongdoing on their part, many officials deny that any such violations even occurred.

The reality is, the COVID-19 pandemic has been very successful in advancing many political and technological pursuits that under normal conditions would have been met with significant barriers.

Prior to their emergency use approval, no nucleic acid vaccines had been licensed for therapeutic use in any country (Croft, 2023, as cited in Dockrell, 2022).[309] Shielded by the perceived emergency, genetic-based vaccines were rushed onto the market, completely bypassing any community-level discussion or debate on the ethics of administering gene-based therapeutics to healthy recipients. Now, with well over 80% of the population having received at least one dose of a genetic vaccine, such a debate almost seems moot. With ethical barriers removed, the door has swung wide open to incorporate mRNA technology into other vaccines and therapeutics, including upcoming annual flu shots.

Both PM Justin Trudeau and his deputy prime minister, Chrystia

Freeland, publicly boasted about how the pandemic provided a great opportunity to accelerate their pre-pandemic efforts on other unrelated fronts and allowed them to usher in policies or programs that under normal circumstances would have encountered substantial pushback.[310] Politicians gained confidence that oppressive tactics will be effective when pursuing other political or ideological agendas, given the massive demonstration of social obedience in the face of flimsy, rather contrived evidence.

We are at a tipping point. Safeguards need to be restored, new ones put in place, and officials held accountable for their decisions, else future restrictions are all but guaranteed. The infrastructure for exploitation has been set and the political desire is certainly there. It is up to the citizens to see to it that it doesn't happen again.

For those who have stood up against the tyranny, you have my deepest gratitude. I can only hope my efforts provide some assistance in the fight.

Thank you for reading.

References

[1] Hart, Robert. "Unvaccinated People Increase Risk of Covid Infection Among Vaccinated, Study Finds." *Forbes*. April 25, 2022. https://www.forbes.com/sites/roberthart/2022/04/25/unvaccinated-people-increase-risk-of-covid-infection-among-vaccinated-study-finds/?sh=3a0da7a124a3.

Lowrie, Morgan. "Mixing with unvaccinated increases COVID-19 risk for vaccinated people, study finds." *The Canadian Press*. April 25, 2022. https://www.cp24.com/news/mixing-with-unvaccinated-increases-covid-19-risk-for-vaccinated-people-study-finds-1.5874637.

[2] Collins English Dictionary. "Fact definition and meaning." Accessed on May 12, 2023. https://www.collinsdictionary.com/dictionary/english/fact.

[3] Merriam-Webster. "Fact Definition & Meaning." Accessed on May 12, 2023. https://www.merriam-webster.com/dictionary/fact.

[4] Altmetric. "Impact of population mixing between vaccinated and unvaccinated subpopulations on infectious disease dynamics: implications for SARS-CoV-2 transmission." Accessed on April 13, 2023. https://cmaj.altmetric.com/details/127235889#score.

[5] University of Toronto Dalla Lana School of Public Health Faculty Database. "Fisman, David N." December 2, 2020. https://www.dlsph.utoronto.ca/faculty-profile/fisman-david-n/.

[6] College of Physicians and Surgeons of Ontario (CPSO). "Fisman, David Norman." Accessed January 16, 2023. https://doctors.cpso.on.ca/DoctorDetails/

Fisman-David-Norman/0062777-75974.

[7] University of Toronto Dalla Lana School of Public Health Faculty Database. "Tuite, Ashleigh." December 4, 2020. https://www.dlsph.utoronto.ca/faculty-profile/tuite-ashleigh/.

[8] Kalvapalle, Rahul. "U of T partners with Moderna to advance research in RNA science and technology." University of Toronto News. April 7, 2022. https://www.utoronto.ca/news/u-t-partners-moderna-advance-research-rna-science-and-technology.

[9] Government of Canada. "Immunization Partnership Fund." November 15, 2022. https://www.canada.ca/en/public-health/services/immunization-vaccine-priorities/immunization-partnership-fund.html#wb-auto-4.

[10] Karl Harrison et Al. v. Attorney General of Canada. Federal Court; Court Number: T-1991-21. Court Files (fct-cf.gc.ca).

Rebel News. "EXCLUSIVE: Top Public Health epidemiologist says vaccine mandates were 'never recommended' for air travel." June 15, 2022. https://www.rebelnews.com/exclusive_top_public_health_epidemiologist_says_vaccine_mandates_were_never_recommended_for_air_travel.

[11] *Macleans*. "The Power List: 50 Canadians who are shaping how we think and live." January 18, 2021. https://www.macleans.ca/rankings/canadas-most-powerful-people-2021/.

[12] University of Toronto, Dalla Lana School of Public Health. "Faculty Database: Fisman, David N." December 2, 2020. https://www.dlsph.utoronto.ca/faculty-profile/fisman-david-n/.

[13] National Collaborating Centre for Infectious Diseases. "Partners: David Fisman." April 28, 2015. https://nccid.ca/partner/david-fisman/.

[14] Ontario Medical Association. Accessed May 6, 2023. https://www.oma.org/expert-advice/request-a-physician-speaker/speakers-search/dr-david-fisman/.

[15] Ontario Medical Association. "OMA Speakers: Dr. David Fisman." Accessed on January 22, 2023. https://www.oma.org/expert-advice/request-a-physician-speaker/speakers-search/dr-david-fisman/.

[16] Vendeville, Geoffrey. "How will the coronavirus spread? U of T epidemiologist deciphers 'messy data'" U of T News. March 6, 2020. https://www.utoronto.ca/news/how-will-coronavirus-spread-u-t-epidemiologist-deciphers-messy-data.

[17] Parliament of Canada. "Evidence - HESA (43-1) - No. 22 - House of Commons of Canada." May 20, 2020. https://www.ourcommons.ca/DocumentViewer/en/43-1/HESA/meeting-22/evidence.

[18] Miller, Adam. "'The time is now to act': COVID-19 spreading in Canada with no known link to travel, previous cases." *CBC News*. March 16, 2020. https://www.cbc.ca/news/health/coronavirus-community-transmission-canada-1.5498804.

[19] Basen, Nathaniel. "COVID-19: The week in review with epidemiologist David Fisman (May 17-22)." *TVO Today.* May 23, 2020. https://www.tvo.org/article/covid-19-the-week-in-review-with-epidemiologist-david-fisman-may-17-22.

[20] CIHR. "Funding Decisions Database." Accessed on May 8, 2023. https://webapps.cihr-irsc.gc.ca/decisions/p/project_details.html?applId=429231&lang=en.

CIHR. "Funding Decisions Database."Accessed on May 8, 2023. https://webapps.cihr-irsc.gc.ca/decisions/p/project_details.html?applId=430473&lang=en.

[21] Basen, Nathaniel. "COVID-19: The week in review with epidemiologist David Fisman." *TVO Today.* April 17, 2020. https://www.tvo.org/article/COVID-19-the-week-in-review-with-epidemiologist-david-fisman.

[22] Furey, Anthony. "Science table member paid by teacher union for arguing against school reopenings; Potential conflict of interest: Expert." *Toronto Sun.* Jan 26, 2021. https://torontosun.com/news/provincial/science-table-member-paid-by-teacher-union-for-arguing-against-school-re-openings.

[23] Sweeney, Ruby. "ETFO suggests schools should stay closed." *BlackburnNews.* January 7, 2021. https://blackburnnews.com/london/london-news/2021/01/07/etfo-suggests-schools-should-stay-closed/.

[24] Science Table, COVID-19 Advisory for Ontario. "Declaration of Interest: David Fisman." February 4, 2021. https://COVID19-sciencetable.ca/wp-content/uploads/2020/07/Declaration-of-Interest_Science-Table_David-Fisman.pdf.

[25] Rodrigues, Gabby. "Ontario COVID-19 science table member resigns after alleging withheld data projects 'grim fall.'" *Global News.* August 23, 2021. https://globalnews.ca/news/8133497/ontario-COVID-science-table-member-resigns-modelling-data/.

[26] Bradley, Jonathan. "U of T professor suggests Conservatives are promoting Nazism." *True North.* August 31, 2021. https://tnc.news/2021/08/31/u-of-t-professor-suggests-conservatives-are-promoting-nazism/.

[27] DeClerq, Katherine. "Ontario COVID-19 science table member resigns, alleges that modelling data 'projects a grim fall'." *CTV News.* August 23, 2021. https://toronto.ctvnews.ca/ontario-covid-19-science-table-member-resigns-alleges-that-modelling-data-projects-a-grim-fall-1.5557510.

Stewart, Ashleigh. "Top epidemiologist resigns from Ontario's COVID-19 science table, alleges withholding of 'grim' projections." *CBC News.* August 23, 2021. https://www.cbc.ca/news/canada/toronto/david-fisman-resignation-covid-science-table-ontario-1.6149961.

[28] Glauser, Wendy. "Mixed messages." *CMAJ.* February 22, 2022 194 (7) E264-E265; DOI: https://doi.org/10.1503/cmaj.1095987.

[29] Ferguson, Rob. "Dr. David Fisman resigns from Ontario's COVID-19 advisory

panel." *The Toronto Star*. August 23, 2021. https://www.thestar.com/politics/provincial/2021/08/23/ontario-science-table-member-dr-david-fisman-resigns-hinting-at-tension-with-other-scientists.html.

[30] Bradley, Jonathan. *True North* (August 31, 2021).

[31] Lilley, Brian. "Court docs show Trudeau's vaccine rules for travel based on politics." *Toronto Sun*. August 10, 2022. https://torontosun.com/opinion/columnists/lilley-court-records-show-trudeau-brought-in-vaccine-mandates-for-travel-purely-based-on-politics.

[32] Elementary Teachers' Federation of Ontario. "ETFO members call for mandatory vaccination of school staff." August 17, 2021. https://www.etfo.ca/news-publications/media-releases/etfo-mandatory-vax.

CISION. "RNAO welcomes continued public health restrictions and mandated vaccination for some health-care workers: More to be done to protect children and economy, nurses say." *Newswire*. August 16, 2021. https://www.newswire.ca/news-releases/rnao-welcomes-continued-public-health-restrictions-and-mandated-vaccination-for-some-health-care-workers-more-to-be-done-to-protect-children-and-economy-nurses-say-826653661.html.

[33] Boisvert, Nick. "Groups representing doctors, nurses call for mandatory vaccination of health-care workers." *CBC News*. August 3, 2021. https://www.cbc.ca/news/politics/cma-cna-mandatory-vaccines-1.6128140.

[34] Romain, Paul L. "Conflicts of interest in research: looking out for number one means keeping the primary interest front and center." *Curr Rev Musculoskelet Med*. June 2015; 8(2): 122–127. doi: 10.1007/s12178-015-9270-2.

De Melo-Martin I, Intemann K. "How do disclosure policies fail? Let us count the ways." *FASEB J*. 2009;23:1638–42. doi: 10.1096/fj.08-125963.

[35] Adamopoulos, Tina. "How should we navigate the next pandemic? U of T researchers are finding the answers." University of Toronto News. November 15, 2022. https://www.utoronto.ca/news/how-should-we-navigate-next-pandemic-u-t-researchers-are-finding-answers.

[36] University of Toronto. "Statement on Research Integrity | Research & Innovation." Accessed on January 20, 2023. https://research.utoronto.ca/research-integrity/statement-research-integrity.

[37] Katz, Gabrielle M. et al. "COVID-19 Vaccine Certificates: Key Considerations for the Ontario Context." Ontario COVID-19 Science Advisory Table. July 21, 2021. https://doi.org/10.47326/ocsat.2021.02.39.1.0.

Faulkner, Harrison. "Ontario Science Table recommends 'vaccine certificates.'" *True North*. July 22, 2021. https://tnc.news/2021/07/22/ontario-science-table-recommends-vaccine-certificates/.

Lilley, Brian. "LILLEY: SciTable wants vax certificates they admit aren't scientific." *Toronto Sun*. July 22, 2021. https://torontosun.com/opinion/columnists/

lilley-science-table-calls-for-vaccine-certificates-they-admit-have-no-scientific-backing.

[38] Freeman, Joshua. "'We're not gonna have a split society': Doug Ford rules out a provincial 'vaccine passport.'" *CTV News*. July 15, 2021. https://toronto.ctvnews.ca/we-re-not-gonna-have-a-split-society-doug-ford-rules-out-a-provincial-vaccine-passport-1.5510704.

[39] Lord, Craig. "Ford supports rapid COVID-19 testing regime for unvaccinated health workers, won't force policy on hospitals." *Global News*. July 26, 2021. https://globalnews.ca/news/8059902/doug-ford-ottawa-covid-announcement-july-26/.

[40] Sitler, Matthew. "Ontario to Require Proof of Vaccination in Select Settings." *Bayshore Broadcasting News Centre*. September 1, 2021. https://www.bayshorebroadcasting.ca/2021/09/01/126846/.

[41] Katz, Gabrielle M. et al. "COVID-19 Vaccine Mandates for Ontario's Hospital Workers: Response to the Premier of Ontario." Ontario COVID-19 Science Advisory Table. October 19, 2021. https://doi.org/10.47326/ocsat.2021.02.49.1.0.

[42] Fox, Chris. "'An evidence-based policy that protects Ontarians:' Science table calls on Ford to mandate vaccines for healthcare workers." *CP24*. October 19, 2021. https://www.cp24.com/news/an-evidence-based-policy-that-protects-ontarians-science-table-calls-on-ford-to-mandate-vaccines-for-healthcare-workers-1.5629724.

[43] Toronto Professional Fire Fighters' Association, I.A.A.F. Local 3888 v Toronto (City), 2022 CanLII 78809 (ON LA), <https://canlii.ca/t/jrpzc>, retrieved on 2023-08-30.

Amalgamated Transit Union, Local 113 v. Toronto Transit Commission, 2021 ONSC 7658. CanLII. https://canlii.ca/t/jklr9. Retrieved on 2023-08-30.

Toronto (City) v Toronto Civic Employees' Union, CUPE, Local 416, 2022 CanLII 109503 (ON LA). https://canlii.ca/t/jt3fv. Retrieved on 2023-08-30.

[44] National Organized Workers Union v Sinai Health System – Affidavit of Dr. Peter Juni. Court File No.: CV-21-671579-0000 Ontario Superior Court of Justice. Sworn November 13, 2021.

[45] Science Table COVID-19 Advisory for Ontario. "Behavioural Science-Informed Strategies for Increasing COVID-19 Vaccine Uptake in Children and Youth: Semantic Scholar." October 26, 2021. https://COVID19-sciencetable.ca/wp-content/uploads/2021/10/Behavioural-Science-Informed-Strategies-for-Increasing-COVID-19-Vaccine-Uptake-in-Children-and-Youth_published_20211026-1.pdf.

[46] Lilley, Brian. "LILLEY: Science Table should disappear and no one should ever mourn it." *Toronto Sun*. August 26, 2022. https://torontosun.com/opinion/columnists/lilley-science-table-should-disappear-and-no-one-should-ever-

mourn-it.

[47] Fox, Chris. "U of T students in residents must be triple vaccinated." *CTV News*. July 29, 2022. https://toronto.ctvnews.ca/u-of-t-students-living-in-residence-will-have-to-be-triple-vaccinated-against-covid-19-1.6007363.

[48] CBC Toronto. "Ontario's top doctor provides update on COVID-19 vaccine booster eligibility, rapid testing program." July 13, 2022. https://www.facebook.com/CBCToronto/videos/3232918990282352/. [25:20 minute mark].

[49] Ziafati, Noushin. "U of T vax policy could boost uptake, but more needed to drive real increase: experts." *CBC News Aug 04, 2022*. https://www.cbc.ca/news/canada/toronto/u-of-t-vax-policy-could-boost-uptake-but-more-needed-to-drive-real-increase-experts-1.6540800.

[50] Fraiman, Joseph, Juan Erviti, Mark Jones, Sander Greenland, Patrick Whelan, Robert M. Kaplan, and Peter Doshi. "Serious adverse events of special interest following mRNA COVID-19 vaccination in randomized trials in adults." *Vaccine* 40(40): 5798–5805. Sept 22, 2022). https://doi.org/10.1016/j.vaccine.2022.08.036.

[51] Mansanguan, Suyanee, Prakaykaew Charunwatthana, Watcharapong Piyaphanee, Wilanee Dechkhajorn, Akkapon Poolcharoen, and Chayasin Mansanguan. "Cardiovascular Manifestation of the BNT162b2 mRNA COVID-19 Vaccine in Adolescents." *Tropical medicine and infectious disease* 7(8):196. Aug 19, 2022. https://doi.org/10.3390/tropicalmed7080196.

[52] Bardosh, Kevin, Allison Krug, Euzebiusz Jamrozik, Trudo Lemmens, Salmaan Keshavjee, Vinay Prasad, Marty A Makary, Stefan Baral, and Tracy Beth Høeg. "COVID-19 vaccine boosters for young adults: a risk benefit assessment and ethical analysis of mandate policies at universities." *BMJ Journal of Medical Ethics*. December 5, 2022. https://jme.bmj.com/content/early/2022/12/05/jme-2022-108449.

[53] Katz, Gabrielle M. et al. "COVID-19 Vaccine Certificates: Key Considerations for the Ontario Context." Ontario COVID-19 Science Advisory Table. July 21, 2021. https://doi.org/10.47326/ocsat.2021.02.39.1.0.

[54] Government of Canada. "Science Shorts 2: The Scientific Method." Accessed on October 11, 2023. https://science.gc.ca/site/science/en/office-chief-science-advisor/resources-and-tools-effective-science-advice/science-shorts-2-scientific-method.

JoVE. "Scientific Method: Steps and Applications – Concept." Accessed on October 11, 2023. https://www.jove.com/science-education/10552/scientific-method-steps-and-applications-concept.

CK-12 Foundation. "Hypothesis." ck12.org. Accessed on October 11, 2023. https://flexbooks.ck12.org/cbook/ck-12-middle-school-physical-science-flexbook-2.0/section/1.19/primary/lesson/hypothesis-ms-ps/.

[55] US Department of Justice, Office of Public Affairs. "Justice Department

Announces Largest Health Care Fraud Settlement in Its History." September 2, 2009. https://www.justice.gov/opa/pr/justice-department-announces-largest-health-care-fraud-settlement-its-history.

[56] US Department of Justice. "Warner-Lambert to pay $430 million to resolve criminal & civil health care liability relating to off-label promotion." USDOJ.GOV. May 13, 2004. https://www.justice.gov/archive/opa/pr/2004/May/04_civ_322.htm.

[57] Ropes & Gray. "DOJ Increases Focus on Clinical Trial Fraud." February 1, 2022. https://www.ropesgray.com/en/newsroom/alerts/2022/february/doj-increases-focus-on-clinical-trial-fraud.

[58] United States Attorney's Office, Western District of Michigan. "Health Care Fraud." Justice.gov. Accessed on December 7, 2022. https://www.justice.gov/usao-wdmi/health-care-fraud.

[59] Canadian Society for the Advancement of Science in Public Policy v Henry, 2022 BCSC 724 at paragraphs 25 & 40. CanLII. https://canlii.ca/t/jp1bz. Retrieved on August 5, 2023.

[60] Behrens, Ralph. "Your Voice: Study on risk of mixing with unvaccinated based on 'unproven and subjective' models." *KelownaNow*. April 29, 2022. https://www.kelownanow.com/watercooler/news/news/COVID_19/Your_Voice_Study_on_risk_of_mixing_with_unvaccinated_based_on_unproven_and_subjective_models/.

[61] Rahhal, Natalie. "Pfizer CEO admits he is 'not certain' their COVID-19 shot will prevent vaccinated people from spreading the virus - as the firm cuts the number of doses it will ship this year." *Daily Mail Online*. December 4, 2020. https://www.dailymail.co.uk/health/article-9018547/Pfizer-CEO-not-certain-COVID-shot-prevents-transmission.html.

[62] Pandolfo, Chris. "Pfizer executive admits COVID-19 vaccine was never tested to prevent transmission: 'This is scandalous'." *The Blaze*. October 11, 2022. https://www.theblaze.com/news/pfizer-executive-admits-COVID-19-vaccine-was-never-tested-to-prevent-transmission-this-is-scandalous.

[63] Palca, Joe. "What A Nasal Spray Vaccine Against COVID-19 Might Do Even Better Than A Shot." *NPR*. August 28, 2020. https://www.npr.org/sections/health-shots/2020/08/28/906797539/what-a-nasal-spray-vaccine-against-COVID-19-might-do-even-better-than-a-shot.

[64] Doshi, Peter. "Will COVID-19 vaccines save lives? Current trials aren't designed to tell us." *BMJ*. October 21, 2020;371:m4037. https://doi.org/10.1136/bmj.m4037.

[65] Pfizer. "FDA Briefing Document Pfizer-BioNTech COVID-19 Vaccine." Vaccines and Related Biological Products Advisory Committee Meeting. December 10, 2020. https://www.fda.gov/media/144245/download.

[66] Polack, Fernando P. et al. "Safety and Efficacy of the BNT162b2 mRNA

COVID-19 Vaccine." *N Engl J Med.* December 31 2020; 383:2603-2615. https://www.nejm.org/doi/10.1056/NEJMoa2034577.

Government of Canada. "Regulatory Decision Summary - COMIRNATY - Health Canada." Canada.ca. September 16, 2021. https://COVID-vaccine.canada.ca/info/regulatory-decision-summary-detail.html?linkID=RDS00856.

Government of Canada. "Regulatory Decision Summary - SPIKEVAX - Health Canada." Canada.ca. September 16, 2021. https://COVID-vaccine.canada.ca/info/regulatory-decision-summary-detail.html?linkID=RDS00855.

[67] Fraiman, Joseph et al. *Vaccine* (September 22, 2022).

[68] UK Health Security Agency. "COVID-19 vaccine surveillance report: week 5, February 3, 2022. London (UK)." UKHSA. 2022. https://assets.publishing.service.gov.uk/government/uploads/system/uploads/attachment_data/file/1052353/Vaccine_surveillance_report_-_week_5.pdf.

Thompson MG, Natarajan K, Irving SA, et al. "Effectiveness of a third dose of mRNA vaccines against COVID-19-associated emergency department and urgent care encounters and hospitalizations among adults during periods of Delta and Omicron variant predominance — VISION Network, 10 states, August 2021–January 2022." *MMWR Morb Mortal Wkly Rep.* 2022;71:139-45. https://doi.org/10.15585/mmwr.mm7104e3.

[69] World Health Organization. "Coronavirus disease (COVID-19): Herd immunity, lockdowns and COVID-19." December 31, 2020. https://www.who.int/news-room/questions-and-answers/item/herd-immunity-lockdowns-and-COVID-19.

Rosove, Jay. "Herd immunity in Alberta: How do we get there, and what if we don't?." *CTV News Edmonton.* March 9, 2021. https://edmonton.ctvnews.ca/herd-immunity-in-alberta-how-do-we-get-there-and-what-if-we-don-t-1.5340515.

Chung, Frank. "Yes, they claimed the vaccines would prevent transmission." *News.com.au.* October 17, 2022. https://www.news.com.au/technology/science/human-body/yes-they-claimed-the-vaccines-would-prevent-transmission/news-story/a176eb002c29e603fc29ef9fe0b33b18.

[70] O'Neill, Natalie. "CDC walks back claim that vaccinated people can't carry COVID-19." *New York Post.* April 2, 2021. https://nypost.com/2021/04/02/cdc-walks-back-claim-that-vaccinated-people-cant-carry-COVID/.

Choi, Joseph. "Fauci: Vaccinated people become 'dead ends' for the coronavirus." *The Hill.* May 16, 2021. https://thehill.com/homenews/sunday-talk-shows/553773-fauci-vaccinated-people-become-dead-ends-for-the-coronavirus/.

[71] Haelle, Tara. "Yes, vaccines block most transmission of COVID-19." *National Geographic.* April 21, 2021. https://www.nationalgeographic.com/science/article/yes-vaccines-block-most-transmission-of-COVID-19.

[72] Tayag, Yasmin. "Why has the CDC stopped collecting data on breakthrough COVID cases?" *The Guardian.* August 6, 2021. https://www.theguardian.com/commentisfree/2021/aug/06/cdc-COVID-coronavirus-data-breakthrough-cases.

[73] UK Health Security Agency. "COVID-19 vaccine surveillance report Week 51." Gov.uk. December 23, 2021. https://assets.publishing.service.gov.uk/government/uploads/system/uploads/attachment_data/file/1043608/Vaccine_surveillance_report_-_week_51.pdf.

Hansen, Christian Holm et al. "Vaccine effectiveness against SARS-CoV-2 infection with the Omicron or Delta variants following a two-dose or booster BNT162b2 or mRNA-1273 vaccination series: A Danish cohort study." *MedRxiv.* January 1, 2021. https://doi.org/10.1101/2021.12.20.21267966.

Lin, Sean and Mingjia Jacky Guan. "'Negative Efficacy' Should Have Stopped COVID Vaccine Recom*mendations in Their Tracks.*" *The Epoch Times.* November 28, 2022. https://www.theepochtimes.com/health/allowing-negative-efficacy-vaccines-upends-pre-pandemic-vaccine-standards_4889548.html.

Brandal Lin T., Emily MacDonald, Lamprini Veneti et al. "Outbreak caused by the SARS-CoV-2 Omicron variant in Norway, November to December 2021." *Eurosurveillance* Volume 26, Issue 50, 16. December 16, 2021. https://doi.org/10.2807/1560-7917.ES.2021.26.50.2101147.

[74] Roth, Asher and Hana Mae Nassar. "'Omicron has been a tsunami': 17M+ Canadians have had Omicron since December." *CityNews.* July 6, 2022. https://vancouver.citynews.ca/2022/07/06/omicron-infections-canada/.

[75] Institute for Health Metrics and Evaluation (IHME). "COVID-19 Results Briefing Canada December 15,2022 Current situation." COVID19.healthdata.org. December 15, 2022. https://www.healthdata.org/sites/default/files/covid_briefs/101_briefing_Canada.pdf.

[76] Ogden NH, Turgeon P, Fazil A, Clark J, Gabriele-Rivet V, Tam T, Ng V. "Counterfactuals of effects of vaccination and public health measures on COVID-19 cases in Canada: What could have happened?" *Can Commun Dis Rep* 2022;48(7/8):292–302. https://doi.org/10.14745/ccdr.v48i78a01.

[77] Watteel, R.N. "Modelers" and their fake simulations need to be reined in, NOW!" Stats Critic. August 26, 2022. https://open.substack.com/pub/statscritic/p/rein-in-modelers?r=1b6bhp&utm_campaign=post&utm_medium=web.

Vickers, David M., John Hardie, Stefan Eberspaecher, Claudia Chaufan and Steven Pelech. "Counterfactuals of effects of vaccination and public health measures on COVID-19 cases in Canada: what could have happened?" *Front. Public Health Sec. Infectious Diseases: Epidemiology and Prevention* Volume 11 – 2023. May 9 2023. https://doi.org/10.3389/fpubh.2023.1173673.

[78] Gilmore, Rachel. "'A big sigh of relief': Trudeau says coronavirus vaccines in spring will begin end of pandemic - National." *Global News.* November 17, 2020.

https://globalnews.ca/news/7467464/coronavirus-trudeau-tough-winter-spring-vaccine/.

[79] D'Mello, Colin, Kayla Goodfield, and Kerrisa Wilson. "Ontario will enter province-wide lockdown as of Christmas Eve, sources say." *CTV News.* December 21, 2020. https://toronto.ctvnews.ca/ontario-will-enter-province-wide-lockdown-as-of-christmas-eve-sources-say-1.5239437.

Harnett, Cindy E. "B.C. restrictions on gatherings to continue through Christmas holidays." *Victoria Times Colonist.* December 7, 2020. https://www.timescolonist.com/local-news/bc-restrictions-on-gatherings-to-continue-through-christmas-holidays-4686082.

Laframboise, Kalina. "Quebec nixes Christmas gatherings as second coronavirus wave gains steam." *Global News.* December 3, 2020. https://globalnews.ca/news/7499664/quebec-christmas-coronavirus-cancelled-gatherings/.

SooToday Staff. "Province extends Reopening Ontario Act orders: Orders extended to February 19." *SooToday.* January 16, 2021. https://www.sootoday.com/local-news/province-extends-reopening-ontario-act-orders-3267398.

Public Safety and Solicitor General. "State of emergency extended to continue B.C.'s COVID-19 response." BC Gov News. February 2, 2021. https://news.gov.bc.ca/releases/2021PSSG0008-000190.

Lowrie, Morgan. "Most COVID-19 restrictions to be extended past February 8, Quebec premier says." *Toronto Star.* January 28, 2021. https://www.thestar.com/politics/2021/01/28/number-of-deaths-jumped-10-per-cent-in-quebec-in-2020-due-to-covid-19-agency-reports.html.

[80] Prime Minister of Canada. "Prime Minister's remarks updating Canadians on the COVID-19 situation and vaccine rollout." Government of Canada. February 5, 2021. https://pm.gc.ca/en/news/speeches/2021/02/05/prime-ministers-remarks-updating-canadians-covid-19-situation-and-vaccine.

[81] Office of the Premier. "Ontario Enacts Provincial Emergency and Stay-at-Home Order: Additional measures needed to protect health system capacity and save lives during third wave of COVID-19." Ontario Newsroom. April 7, 2021. https://news.ontario.ca/en/release/61029/ontario-enacts-provincial-emergency-and-stay-at-home-order.

Jenner, Catherine and Andrew Cunningham. "Québec's Regional And Province-Wide Restrictions In Response To COVID-19 Resurgence - Operational Impacts and Strategy - Canada." *Mondaq.* April 28, 2021. https://www.mondaq.com/canada/operational-impacts-and-strategy/1062266/qubec39s-regional-and-province-wide-restrictions-in-response-to-covid-19-resurgence.

Public Safety and Solicitor General. "Province introduces travel restrictions to curb spread of COVID-19." BC Gov News. April 23, 2021. https://news.gov.bc.ca/releases/2021PSSG0029-000758.

[82] Taylor, Brooke. "Cycles of lockdown and doubt: Canada's way out of COVID-19 pandemic depends on vaccines, expert says." *CTV News*. April 08, 2021. https://www.ctvnews.ca/health/coronavirus/cycles-of-lockdown-and-doubt-canada-s-way-out-of-covid-19-pandemic-depends-on-vaccines-expert-says-1.5379072.

[83] Orton, Tyler. "'Freer' and 'more normal' summer possible if 70% of Canadians get first dose: Trudeau." *Business in Vancouver*. May 11, 2021. https://biv.com/article/2021/05/freer-and-more-normal-summer-possible-if-70-canadians-get-first-dose-trudeau.

[84] World Health Organization. "Achieving 70% COVID-19 Immunization Coverage by Mid-2022." December 23 2021. https://www.who.int/news/item/23-12-2021-achieving-70-covid-19-immunization-coverage-by-mid-2022.

OECD. "Access to COVID-19 vaccines: Global approaches in a global crisis." March 18 2021. https://www.oecd.org/coronavirus/policy-responses/access-to-covid-19-vaccines-global-approaches-in-a-global-crisis-c6a18370/.

[85] Goldstein, Lorrie. "GOLDSTEIN: Even Trudeau knows targeting unvaccinated un-Canadian." *Toronto Sun*. January 08, 2022. https://torontosun.com/opinion/columnists/goldstein-even-trudeau-knows-targeting-unvaccinated-un-canadian.

[86] Tasker, John Paul. "Canada has ordered more than 400 million COVID-19 vaccine shots: Here's the progress report." *CBC News*. May 26, 2021. https://www.cbc.ca/news/politics/canada-vaccine-deliveries-progress-report-1.6034624.

[87] Government of Canada. "Procuring vaccines for COVID-19." Canada.ca. Accessed on January 21, 2023. https://www.canada.ca/en/public-services-procurement/services/procuring-vaccines-covid19.html#agreements.

[88] Tasker, John Paul. "Trudeau promises $1B to help provinces pay for vaccine passports." *CBC News*. August 27, 2021. https://www.cbc.ca/news/politics/trudeau-promises-1b-vaccine-passports-1.6155618.

[89] Moderna. "FDA Briefing Document: Moderna COVID-19 Vaccine." Vaccines and Related Biological Products Advisory Committee Meeting. December 17, 2020. https://www.fda.gov/media/144434/download.

Pfizer. "FDA Briefing Document Pfizer-BioNTech COVID-19 Vaccine." Vaccines and Related Biological Products Advisory Committee Meeting. December 10, 2020. https://www.fda.gov/media/144245/download.

[90] Lovelace, Berkeley Jr. "CDC study shows 74% of people infected in Massachusetts Covid outbreak were fully vaccinated." *CNBC*. July 31, 2021. https://www.cnbc.com/2021/07/30/cdc-study-shows-74percent-of-people-infected-in-massachusetts-covid-outbreak-were-fully-vaccinated.html.

[91] Brown CM, Vostok J, Johnson H, et al. "Outbreak of SARS-CoV-2 Infections,

Including COVID-19 Vaccine Breakthrough Infections, Associated with Large Public Gatherings — Barnstable County, Massachusetts, July 2021." *MMWR Morb Mortal Wkly Rep* 2021;70:1059-1062. http://dx.doi.org/10.15585/mmwr.mm7031e2.

[92] Frantzman, Seth J. "Lessons, cautionary tales from Israel on the pandemic's next stage." *The Jerusalem Post.* July 31, 2021. https://www.jpost.com/opinion/lessons-cautionary-tale-from-israel-on-the-pandemics-next-stage-675465.

[93] Our World in Data. "Coronavirus (COVID-19) Vaccinations." Accessed on July 17, 2023. https://ourworldindata.org/covid-vaccinations.

[94] Goldberg, Yair, Micha Mandel, Yinon M Bar-On et al. "Waning Immunity after the BNT162b2 Vaccine in Israel." *N Engl J Med.* December 9 2021;385(24):e85. doi: https://doi.org/10.1056/NEJMoa2114228. Epub 2021 Oct 27.

[95] Avis, Daniel. "Israel's COVID-19 surge shows the world what's coming next." *National Post.* September 7, 2021. https://nationalpost.com/news/world/israels-covid-19-surge-shows-the-world-whats-coming-next.

[96] Prime Minister of Canada. "Prime Minister announces mandatory vaccination for the federal workforce and federally regulated transportation sectors." Government of Canada. October 6, 2021. https://pm.gc.ca/en/news/news-releases/2021/10/06/prime-minister-announces-mandatory-vaccination-federal-workforce-and.

[97] Zuber, Melissa Couto. "'Waning immunity?' Some experts say term leads to false understanding of COVID-19 vaccines." *CBC News.* September 19, 2021. https://www.cbc.ca/news/health/waning-immunity-some-experts-say-term-leads-to-false-understanding-of-covid-19-vaccines-1.6181637.

Miller, Adam. "Why 'waning immunity' from COVID-19 vaccines isn't as bad as it sounds." *CBC News.* October 23, 2021. https://www.cbc.ca/news/health/waning-immunity-covid-19-vaccines-breakthrough-infections-canada-1.6221608.

AstraZeneca. "Waning immunity and the role of booster vaccinations." October 5 2021. https://www.astrazeneca.com/what-science-can-do/topics/covid-19/waning-immunity.html.

[98] Smyth, Jamie. "Moderna chief predicts existing vaccines will struggle with Omicron." *Financial Times.* November 30, 2021. https://www.ft.com/content/27def1b9-b9c8-47a5-8e06-72e432e0838f.

Brooks, Khristopher J. "Moderna's CEO says current COVID-19 vaccines likely won't work as well against Omicron." *CBS News.* December 1, 2021. https://www.cbsnews.com/news/covid-omicron-variant-vaccine-moderna/.

[99] Davies, Pascale. "Omicron: 3 vaccine doses are not enough to stop the new COVID variant, warns BioNTech CEO." *Euronews.* December 20, 2021. https://www.euronews.com/next/2021/12/20/omicron-3-vaccine-doses-are-not-enough-to-stop-the-new-covid-variant-warns-biontech-ceo.

[100] Office of the Premier. "Ontario Temporarily Moving to Modified Step Two of the Roadmap to Reopen: Time-limited measures needed to preserve hospital capacity as province continues to accelerate booster dose rollout." Ontario Newsroom. January 3, 2022. https://news.ontario.ca/en/release/1001394/ontario-temporarily-moving-to-modified-step-two-of-the-roadmap-to-reopen.

Martins, Nikitha. "B.C. adding COVID-19 restrictions as booster rollout, rapid testing accelerates." *CityNews*. December 21, 2021. https://vancouver.citynews.ca/2021/12/21/bc-covid-restrictions-booster-rapid-test/.

Stikeman Elliott LLP. "Québec Modifies Restrictions as of January 17 and 24, 2022: No Curfew, No Sunday Closures but Vaccine Passport extended to SAQs, SQDCs, Big Box Stores." Stikeman.com. January 17, 2022. https://www.jdsupra.com/legalnews/quebec-modifies-restrictions-as-of-8939989/.

[101] Zimonjic, Peter. "Provinces could make vaccination mandatory, says federal health minister." *CBC News*. January 7, 2022. https://www.cbc.ca/news/politics/duclos-mandatory-vaccination-policies-on-way-1.6307398.

[102] Zimonjic, Peter. "Trudeau says Canadians are 'angry' and 'frustrated' with the unvaccinated." *CBC News*. January 5, 2022. https://www.cbc.ca/news/politics/trudeau-unvaccinated-canadians-covid-hospitals-1.6305159.

[103] Government of Canada. "Requirements for truckers entering Canada in effect as of January 15, 2022." Canada.ca. January 13, 2022. https://www.canada.ca/en/public-health/news/2022/01/requirements-for-truckers-entering-canada-in-effect-as-of-january-15-2022.html.

[104] Gunter, Lorne. "GUNTER: Roll on, Freedom Convoy." *Ottawa Sun*. Jan 25, 2022. https://ottawasun.com/opinion/columnists/gunter-roll-on-freedom-convoy/wcm/fc6c6382-0d87-48bc-81c4-2cd89bc4d97c.

Wikipedia. "Timeline of the Canada convoy protest." Accessed on Dec. 26, 2022. https://en.wikipedia.org/wiki/Timeline_of_the_Canada_convoy_protest.

[105] Campbell, Neil. "Canadian Provinces Begin Relenting on Mandates Amidst Ongoing Freedom Convoy Protests." *Vision Times*. February 09, 2022. https://www.visiontimes.com/2022/02/09/canada-drops-vaccine-passports-mask-mandates.html.

CBC News. "Coronavirus Brief." Feb. 15, 2022. https://subscriptions.cbc.ca/newsletter_static/messages/coronavirusbrief/2022-02-15/.

[106] Wolfe, Tobin. "Vaccine Passports Ending in 9 Provinces." *The Canadian Dissident*. March 1, 2022. http://www.canadiandissident.ca/2022/03/vaccine-passports-ending-in-9-provinces.html.

[107] Shield, David. "Sask. premier plans to scrap proof of vaccination requirement by end of February." *CBC News*. February 1, 2022. https://www.cbc.ca/news/canada/saskatoon/sask-premier-plans-to-scrap-proof-of-vaccination-requirement-by-end-of-february-1.6334882.

[108] Moe, Scott. "A message from Premier Scott Moe." Twitter. January 29, 2022. https://twitter.com/PremierScottMoe/status/1487460075102871554.

[109] Tunney, Catharine. "Federal government invokes Emergencies Act for first time ever in response to protests, blockades." *CBC News*. February 14, 2022. https://www.cbc.ca/news/politics/trudeau-premiers-cabinet-1.6350734.

[110] Public Order Emergency Commission (POEC). "Public Hearing." Volume 30. November 24, 2022. https://publicorderemergencycommission.ca/files/documents/Transcripts/POEC-Public-Hearings-Volume-30-November-24-2022.pdf.

[111] Anthes, Emily. "Booster protection wanes against symptomatic Omicron infections, British data suggests: A new study found that booster protection against symptomatic Omicron fades within 10 weeks." *The New York Times*. December 23, 2021. https://www.nytimes.com/2021/12/23/health/booster-protection-omicron.html.

[112] Joy, Lisa. "Federal Court documents reveal travel ban not based on science." *SaskToday.ca*. Aug 15, 2022. https://www.sasktoday.ca/north/local-news/federal-court-documents-reveal-travel-ban-not-based-on-science-5700885.

Subramanya, Rupa. "Court Documents Reveal Canada's Travel Ban Had No Scientific Basis." *The Free Press*. August 2, 2022. https://www.thefp.com/p/court-documents-reveal-canadas-travel.

[113] Razak, Fahad, Saeha Shin, C. David Naylor and Arthur S. Slutsky. "Canada's response to the initial 2 years of the COVID-19 pandemic: a comparison with peer countries." *CMAJ*. June 27, 2022: 194 (25) E870-E877. https://doi.org/10.1503/cmaj.220316; https://www.cmaj.ca/content/194/25/E870.

[114] Hall, Chris. "Trudeau defends vax mandates, Emergencies Act decision, in interview." *CBC News*. June 24, 2022. https://www.cbc.ca/news/politics/trudeau-vax-mandates-emergency-act-1.6499214.

[115] Dzsurdzsa, Cosmin. "Health Canada considering recommending a booster every three months." *True North*. September 2, 2022. https://tnc.news/2022/09/02/health-canada-booster/.

[116] Government of Canada. "Health Canada authorizes first bivalent COVID-19 booster for adults 18 years and older." Canada.ca. September 1, 2022. https://www.canada.ca/en/health-canada/news/2022/09/health-canada-authorizes-first-bivalent-covid-19-booster-for-adults-18-years-and-older.html.

[117] Miller, Adam. "Moderna is banking on a combined COVID, flu and RSV vaccine. Will it work?:Controversial decision to promote shot before clinical trials are done raises concerns." *CBC News*. Nov 12, 2022. https://www.cbc.ca/news/health/moderna-covid-flu-rsv-vaccine-1.6647447.

[118] Ontario Ministry of Health. "COVID-19 Vaccine Booster Recommendations." August 31, 2022. https://www.health.gov.on.ca/en/pro/programs/publichealth/

coronavirus/docs/vaccine/COVID-19_vaccine_third_dose_ recommendations.pdf.

[119] Public Health Ontario. "Surveillance Report: COVID-19 Vaccine Uptake in Ontario: December 14, 2020 to January 15, 2023." Accessed January 21, 2023. Publichealthontario.ca. https://www.publichealthontario.ca/-/media/documents/ ncov/epi/covid-19-vaccine-uptake-ontario-epi-summary.pdf.

[120] Johns Hopkins Coronavirus Resource Center. "Vaccine Research & Development." January 22, 2023. https://coronavirus.jhu.edu/vaccines/timeline.

World Economic Forum. "5 charts that tell the story of vaccines today." June 2, 2020. https://www.weforum.org/agenda/2020/06/vaccine-development-barriers-coronavirus/.

[121] Government of Canada. "Health Canada Decision-Making Framework for Identifying, Assessing, and Managing Health Risks - August 1, 2000." Accessed on January 22, 2023. https://www.canada.ca/en/health-canada/corporate/about-health-canada/reports-publications/health-products-food-branch/health-canada-decision-making-framework-identifying-assessing-managing-health-risks.html#a35.

Government of Canada. "Format and content for post-market drug benefit-risk assessment in Canada - Guidance document." Accessed on January 22, 2023. https://www.canada.ca/en/health-canada/services/publications/drugs-health-products/content-drug-benefit-risk-assessment/guidance-document.html#a1.3.1.

House of Commons of Canada. "Committee Report No. 7 - HESA (39-2)." Accessed on January 22, 2023. https://www.ourcommons.ca/DocumentViewer/ en/39-2/HESA/report-7/page-69.

[122] CPSA. "Further action to address the spread of COVID-19 misinformation by physicians - College of Physicians & Surgeons of Alberta." October 14, 2021. https://cpsa.ca/news/further-action-to-address-the-spread-of-covid-19-misinformation-by-physicians/.

Stewart, Ashleigh. "40 Ontario physicians currently being investigated for COVID-19 issues: College." *Global News.* January 20, 2022. https://globalnews.ca/ news/8524589/ontario-physicians-investigation-covid-19/.

[123] Radcliffe, Shawn. "The Future of Vaccines: Could mRNA Revolutionize Disease Prevention?" *Healthline.* Accessed on January 23, 2022. https:// transform.healthline.com/future-of-health/could-mrna-technology-revolutionize-future-vaccines-and-treatments.

[124] Goldfarb, Theodore D. and Michael S. Pritchard. "Overly Ambitious Researchers - Fabricating Data." Online Ethics Center (2000). Accessed on January 24, 2023. https://onlineethics.org/cases/ethics-science-classroom/ overly-ambitious-researchers-fabricating-data.

[125] Northern Illinois University. "Fabrication or Falsification | Academic Integrity

Tutorial for Students." Accessed May 31, 2022. (niu.edu) https://www.niu.edu/academic-integrity/students/cheating/fabrication-or-falsification.shtml.

[126] Kuali. "The Importance of Taking Research Misconduct Seriously." Accessed on May 31, 2022. https://www.kuali.co/post/research-misconduct-why-we-need-to-take-it-seriously.

[127] Schank, Eric. "Merely hanging out with unvaccinated people puts the vaccinated at higher risk: study." *Salon*. April 27, 2022. https://www.salon.com/2022/04/27/unvaccinated-risk/.

[128] Hart, Robert. "Unvaccinated People Increase Risk of Covid Infection Among Vaccinated, Study Finds." *Forbes*. April 25, 2022. https://www.forbes.com/sites/roberthart/2022/04/25/unvaccinated-people-increase-risk-of-covid-infection-among-vaccinated-study-finds/?sh=3a0da7a124a3.

[129] Henderson, Emily. "Unvaccinated people threaten the safety of individuals vaccinated against SARS-CoV-2." *News Medical*. April 25, 2022. https://www.news-medical.net/news/20220425/Unvaccinated-people-threaten-the-safety-of-individuals-vaccinated-against-SARS-CoV-2.aspx.

[130] Woo, Andrea. "Unvaccinated disproportionately risk safety of those vaccinated against COVID-19, study shows." *Globe and Mail*. April 25, 2022. https://www.theglobeandmail.com/canada/article-unvaccinated-covid-risk-for-vaccinated-canada/.

[131] Ellis, Ralph. "Unvaccinated People Create Higher Risk for Vaccinated, Study Says." *WebMD*. April 27, 2022. https://www.webmd.com/vaccines/covid-19-vaccine/news/20220427/unvaccinated-people-create-higher-risk-for-vaccinated-study-says.

[132] *Healthline*. "Study: Unvaccinated People Increase COVID-19 Risk, Even Among Vaccinated People." April 25, 2022. https://www.healthline.com/health-news/study-unvaccinated-people-increase-covid-19-risk-even-among-vaccinated-people.

[133] Lavery, Irelyne. "Unvaccinated people increase risk of COVID-19 infection among vaccinated: study." *Global News*. April 25, 2022. https://globalnews.ca/news/8783380/unvaccinated-vaccinated-covid-risk-canadian-study/. [Video] https://youtu.be/SDefEK6PDg0.

[134] Lowrie, Morgan. "Mixing with the unvaccinated increases COVID-19 risk for the vaccinated, study finds." *Canadian Press*. April 25, 2022. https://www.cp24.com/news/mixing-with-unvaccinated-increases-covid-19-risk-for-vaccinated-people-study-finds-1.5874637?cache=m.

[135] Lowrie, Morgan. "Mixing with the unvaccinated increases COVID-19 risk for the vaccinated, study finds." *Toronto Sun*. April 25, 2022. https://torontosun.com/health/mixing-with-the-unvaccinated-increases-covid-19-risk-for-the-vaccinated-study-finds.

[136] Lowrie, Morgan. "Mixing with the unvaccinated increases COVID-19 risk for the vaccinated, study finds." *Vancouver Sun.* April 25, 2022. https://vancouversun.com/health/mixing-with-the-unvaccinated-increases-covid-19-risk-for-the-vaccinated-study-finds/wcm/fa162793-c586-4717-9150-8d3e0fe8d43c.

[137] Lowrie, Morgan. "Mixing with the unvaccinated increases COVID-19 risk for the vaccinated, study finds." *Calgary Sun.* April 25, 2022. https://calgarysun.com/health/mixing-with-the-unvaccinated-increases-covid-19-risk-for-the-vaccinated-study-finds/wcm/91c3292a-99a6-44f3-95e5-0b2cdc612a1a.

[138] Lowrie, Morgan. "Mixing with the unvaccinated increases COVID-19 risk for the vaccinated, study finds." *Toronto Star.* April 25, 2022. https://www.thestar.com/news/canada/2022/04/25/mixing-with-unvaccinated-increases-covid-19-risk-for-vaccinated-people-study-finds.html.

[139] Lowrie, Morgan. "Mixing with the unvaccinated increases COVID-19 risk for the vaccinated, study finds." *Montreal Gazette.* April 25, 2022. https://montrealgazette.com/pmn/news-pmn/canada-news-pmn/mixing-with-unvaccinated-increases-covid-19-risk-for-vaccinated-people-study-finds-2/wcm/964efac0-7226-46c2-b546-2e4c57d7e036.

[140] Lowrie, Morgan. "Mixing with the unvaccinated increases COVID-19 risk for the vaccinated, study finds." *National Observer.* April 25, 2022. https://www.nationalobserver.com/2022/04/25/news/mixing-unvaccinated-risk-covid-vaccinated.

[141] Lowrie, Morgan. "Mixing with the unvaccinated increases COVID-19 risk for the vaccinated, study finds." *National Post.* April 25, 2022. https://nationalpost.com/pmn/news-pmn/canada-news-pmn/mixing-with-unvaccinated-increases-covid-19-risk-for-vaccinated-people-study-finds.

[142] Lowrie, Morgan. "Mixing with the unvaccinated increases COVID-19 risk for the vaccinated, study finds." *CTV News.* April 25, 2022. https://www.ctvnews.ca/health/coronavirus/being-with-unvaccinated-people-increases-covid-19-risk-for-those-who-are-vaccinated-modelling-study-1.5874632.

[143] Lowrie, Morgan. "Mixing with the unvaccinated increases COVID-19 risk for the vaccinated, study finds." *The Chronicle Journal.* April 25, 2022. https://www.chroniclejournal.com/news/national/mixing-with-unvaccinated-increases-covid-19-risk-for-vaccinated-people-study-finds/article_16559b81-d081-5d4a-9756-7ae399873fd5.html.

[144] Lowrie, Morgan. "Mixing with the unvaccinated increases COVID-19 risk for the vaccinated, study finds." *Canoe.com.* April 25, 2022. https://canoe.com/diseases-and-conditions/coronavirus/vaccine-for-coronavirus/mixing-with-unvaccinated-increases-covid-19-risk-for-vaccinated-people-study.

[145] Lowrie, Morgan. "Mixing with the unvaccinated increases COVID-19 risk for the vaccinated, study finds." *OHS Canada.* April 25, 2022. https://

www.ohscanada.com/mixing-with-unvaccinated-increases-covid-19-risk-for-vaccinated-people-study-finds/.

[146] Lowrie, Morgan. "Mixing with the unvaccinated increases COVID-19 risk for the vaccinated, study finds." *Prince George Citizen.* April 25, 2022. https://www.princegeorgecitizen.com/national-news/mixing-with-unvaccinated-increases-covid-19-risk-for-vaccinated-people-study-finds-5295746.

[147] Lowrie, Morgan. "Mixing with the unvaccinated increases COVID-19 risk for the vaccinated, study finds." *The Abbotsford News.* April 25, 2022. https://www.abbynews.com/news/mixing-with-unvaccinated-increases-covid-19-risk-for-vaccinated-people-study-finds/.

[148] Lowrie, Morgan. "Mixing with the unvaccinated increases COVID-19 risk for the vaccinated, study finds." *The Williams Lake Tribune.* April 25, 2022. https://www.wltribune.com/news/mixing-with-unvaccinated-increases-covid-19-risk-for-vaccinated-people-study-finds/.

[149] Lowrie, Morgan. "Mixing with the unvaccinated increases COVID-19 risk for the vaccinated, study finds." *The Edmonton Journal.* April 25, 2022. https://edmontonjournal.com/news/national/mixing-with-unvaccinated-increases-covid-19-risk-for-vaccinated-people-study-finds/wcm/658033d5-4aa5-43e7-b227-36e0e4a53a00/amp/.

[150] Lowrie, Morgan. "Mixing with the unvaccinated increases COVID-19 risk for the vaccinated, study finds." *Richmond News.* April 25, 2022. https://www.richmond-news.com/national-news/mixing-with-unvaccinated-increases-covid-19-risk-for-vaccinated-people-study-finds-5295746.

[151] Lowrie, Morgan. "Mixing with the unvaccinated increases COVID-19 risk for the vaccinated, study finds." *The Chilliwack Progress.* April 25, 2022. https://www.theprogress.com/news/mixing-with-unvaccinated-increases-covid-19-risk-for-vaccinated-people-study-finds/.

[152] Lowrie, Morgan. "Mixing with the unvaccinated increases COVID-19 risk for the vaccinated, study finds." *MYMcMurray.com.* April 25, 2022. https://www.mymcmurray.com/2022/04/25/mixing-with-unvaccinated-increases-covid-19-risk-for-vaccinated-people-study-finds/.

[153] Lowrie, Morgan. "Mixing with the unvaccinated increases COVID-19 risk for the vaccinated, study finds." *Castanet.net.* April 25, 2022. https://www.castanet.net/news/Canada/366935/Mixing-with-unvaccinated-increases-COVID-19-risk-for-vaccinated-people-study-finds.

[154] Ranger, Michael. "Mixing with unvaccinated increases COVID-19 risk for vaccinated: Study." *CityNews Everywhere.* April 25, 2022. https://toronto.citynews.ca/2022/04/25/covid-19-unvaccinated-vaccinated-study/.

[155] Pandey, Kirti. "Study shows mixing with unvaccinated people poses risk of contracting SARS-CoV-2 infection in vaccinated persons." *TimesNowNews India.*

April 25, 2022. https://www.timesnownews.com/health/study-shows-mixing-with-unvaccinated-people-poses-risk-of-contracting-sars-cov-2-infection-in-vaccinated-persons-article-91075728.

[156] *Scimex.* "The unvaccinated increase the risk of COVID-19 for the vaccinated when they mingle." *Science Media Exchange – Scimex Breaking science news for Australia & New Zealand.* April 25, 2022. https://www.scimex.org/newsfeed/unvaccinated-people-put-vaccinated-people-at-higher-covid-19-risk-when-they-mingle.

[157] Frketich, Joanna. "Unvaxxed pose risk of infection for those with shots, research shows as wastewaster suggests COVID soars in Hamilton." *The Hamilton Spectator.* April 26, 2022. https://www.thespec.com/news/hamilton-region/2022/04/26/covid-19-hamilton-latest-news.html.

[158] Johnson, Kate. "My Choice? Unvaccinated Pose Outsize Risk to Vaccinated." *Medscape Medical News.* May 10, 2022. https://www.medscape.com/viewarticle/973711.

[159] Fisman, David N. Twitter (@DFisman). July 22, 2021.

[160] Katz, Gabrielle M. et al. OCSAT (July 21, 2021).

[161] Constitutional Rights Centre. "Statement of Claim Between Dr. Byram Bridle and University of Guelph, Jeffrey Wichtel, Laurie Arnott, Charlotte Yates, Scott Weese, Glen Pyle, Andrew Peregrine, Dorothee Bienzle, Amy Greer, David Fisman, Nick Duley, Jane or John Doe Junior Scientist: Court File No./N° du dossier du greffe: CV-22-00691880-0000." December 19, 2022. https://www.constitutionalrightscentre.ca/20CRC16/wp-content/uploads/2022/12/ISSUED-SOC-ByramBridle.pdf.

[162] Fisman, David N. Twitter (@DFisman). June 9, 2021.

[163] House of Commons of Canada. "Debates (Hansard) No. 61 - April 29, 2022 (44-1)." April 29, 2022. https://www.ourcommons.ca/DocumentViewer/en/44-1/house/sitting-61/hansard.

[164] UKHSA. "COVID-19 vaccine quarterly surveillance reports (Jan 2022 to March 2022)." GOV.UK. Accessed on July 17, 2023. https://www.gov.uk/government/publications/covid-19-vaccine-weekly-surveillance-reports.

[165] Nabin K Shrestha et al. "Effectiveness of the Coronavirus Disease 2019 Bivalent Vaccine." *Open Forum Infectious Diseases*, Volume 10, Issue 6. June 2023, ofad209, https://doi.org/10.1093/ofid/ofad209.

[166] Fenton, Norman. "The vaccine efficacy illusion revisited." YouTube. May 1, 2023. https://www.youtube.com/watch?v=Gkh6N-ZL3_k.

[167] Fisman, David N. Twitter (@DFisman). July 22, 2021.

[168] Bardosh, Kevin, Allison Krug, Euzebiusz Jamrozik, Trudo Lemmens, Salmaan Keshavjee, Vinay Prasad, Marty A Makary, Stefan Baral, and Tracy Beth Høeg. "COVID-19 vaccine

boosters for young adults: a risk benefit assessment and ethical analysis of mandate policies at universities." *Journal of Medical Ethics.* December 5, 2022. https://jme.bmj.com/content/early/2022/12/05/jme-2022-108449.

[169] Miltimore, Jon. "England Refuses to Offer COVID Shots to Kids Under 12, While US Cities Mandate Them. Who's Right?: Jon Miltimore." *FEE Freeman Article.* September 14, 2022. https://fee.org/articles/england-refuses-to-offer-covid-shots-to-kids-under-12-while-us-cities-mandate-them-who-s-right/.

[170] Goldenberg, Joel. "Denmark halts COVID vaccinations for low-risk people under 50." *The Suburban Newspaper.* September 16, 2022. https://www.thesuburban.com/news/city_news/denmark-halts-covid-vaccinations-for-low-risk-people-under-50/article_1e0264ec-dea3-59e0-bf3e-db59eee4378d.html.

[171] Collier, Roger. "Scientific misconduct or criminal offence?" *CMAJ.* November 17, 2015 187 (17) 1273-1274. https://doi.org/10.1503/cmaj.109-5171.

[172] Bhutta, Zulfiqar and Julian Crane. "Should research fraud be a crime?" *BMJ.* July 15, 2014; 349 doi: https://doi.org/10.1136/bmj.g4532.

Harvey, Lee. "Research fraud: a long-term problem exacerbated by the clamour for research grants." *Quality in Higher Education.* October 28, 2020 (Volume 26, 2020 - Issue 3). https://doi.org/10.1080/13538322.2020.1820126.

[173] United States House Committee on Oversight and Accountability. "Because I Said So: Examining the Science and Impact of COVID-19 Vaccine Mandates [Video 1:35:15 and 2:03:30 min marks]." July 27, 2023. https://oversight.house.gov/hearing/because-i-said-so-examining-the-science-and-impact-of-covid-19-vaccine-mandates/.

[174] Karl Harrison et Al. v. Attorney General of Canada. Federal Court; Court Number: T-1991-21. Court Files (fct-cf.gc.ca).

[175] Joy, Lisa. "Federal Court documents reveal travel ban not based on science." *SaskToday.ca.* Aug 15, 2022. https://www.sasktoday.ca/north/local-news/federal-court-documents-reveal-travel-ban-not-based-on-science-5700885.

[176] Rebel News. "EXCLUSIVE: Top Public Health epidemiologist says vaccine mandates were 'never recommended' for air travel." June 15, 2022. https://www.rebelnews.com/exclusive_top_public_health_epidemiologist_says_vaccine_mandates_were_never_recommended_for_air_travel.

[177] Public Order Emergency Commission (POEC). "Public Hearing." Volume 30. November 24, 2022. https://publicorderemergencycommission.ca/files/documents/Transcripts/POEC-Public-Hearings-Volume-30-November-24-2022.pdf.

[178] Risdon, Melanie. "Calgary medical specialist and lawyer refute misinformation on unvaxxed being COVID spreaders: Calgary pediatrician Dr. Eric Payne and lawyer Jeff Rath of Rath & Company, join the Western Standard's Melanie Risdon to discuss a recent study released by David Fisman

indicating unvaccinated individuals pose an increased risk of transmitting COVID-19 to those vaccinated." *Western Standard*. April 28, 2022. https://www.facebook.com/watch/live/?ref=watch_permalink&v=721575942194974.

[179] CMAJ. "Impact of population mixing between vaccinated and unvaccinated subpopulations on infectious disease dynamics: implications for SARS-CoV-2 transmission." Accessed on June 22, 2022. https://www.cmaj.ca/content/194/16/E573/tab-e-letters.

[180] Bridle, Byram W. "Fiction Disguised as Science to Promote Hatred: Disinformation Must Be Called Out." COVID Chronicles. April 27, 2022. https://viralimmunologist.substack.com/p/fiction-disguised-as-science-to-promote.

[181] Horwood, Matthew. "Critics say widely shared study on mixing with unvaccinated 'contain massive errors.'" Western Standard. April 28, 2022. https://www.westernstandard.news/news/critics-say-widely-shared-study-on-mixing-with-unvaccinated-contain-massive-errors/article_f5f1d4a4-a11a-575c-9ba8-1c2c24e8eaae.html.

[182] Rose, Jessica. "Call for retraction of paper entitled: "Impact of population mixing between vaccinated and unvaccinated subpopulations on infectious disease dynamics: implications for SARS-CoV-2 transmission." Unacceptable Jessica. Apr 28, 2022. https://open.substack.com/pub/jessicar/p/call-for-retraction-of-paper-entitled?r=1b6bhp&utm_campaign=post&utm_medium=web.

[183] Fisman, David N., Afia Amoako, and Ashleigh R. Tuite. "(Preprint v1) Impact of Population Mixing Between a Vaccinated Majority and Unvaccinated Minority on Disease Dynamics: Implications for SARS-CoV-2." *ResearchGate*. December 16, 2021. https://www.researchgate.net/publication/357105454_Impact_of_Population_Mixing_Between_a_Vaccinated_Majority_and_Unvaccinated_Minority_on_Disease_Dynamics_Implications_for_SARS-CoV-2.

[184] Fisman, David N., Afia Amoako, and Ashleigh R. Tuite. "(Preprint v2) Impact of Population Mixing Between a Vaccinated Majority and Unvaccinated Minority on Disease Dynamics: Implications for SARS-CoV-2." *ResearchGate*. March 4, 2022. https://doi.org/10.1101/2021.12.14.21267742.

[185] Fisman, David N., Afia Amoako, Ashleigh R. Tuite. "Impact of population mixing between vaccinated and unvaccinated subpopulations on infectious disease dynamics: implications for SARS-CoV-2 transmission." *CMAJ*. April 25, 2022;194:E573-E580. https://doi.org/10.1503/cmaj.212105.

[186] Canadian Medical Association Journal. "CMAJ Editorial Independence." Accessed on January 22, 2023. https://www.cma.ca/about-cma/cmaj-editorial-independence.

[187] Patrick, Kirsten. "Countering more virulent SARS-CoV-2 variants will require a smarter pandemic response." *CMAJ*. October 25, 2021 193 (42) E1633-E1634. https://doi.org/10.1503/cmaj.211656.

[188] McRae, Andrew D. and Andreas Laupacis. "SARS-CoV-2 vaccination should be required to practise medicine in Canada." *CMAJ*. November 29, 2021 193 (47) E1816-E1817. https://doi.org/10.1503/cmaj.211839.

[189] The Governor General of Canada. "Order of Canada appointees – December 2022." gg.ca. Accessed on January 5, 2023. https://www.gg.ca/en/order-canada-appointees-december-2022.

[190] Fisman, David N., Afia Amoako, Allison Simmons and Ashleigh R. Tuite. "(preprint) Impact of Immune Evasion, Waning and Boosting on Dynamics of Population Mixing Between a Vaccinated Majority and Unvaccinated Minority." *MedRxiv*. February 7 2023. https://doi.org/10.1101/2023.02.03.23285437.

[191] Karen Wallace, Email correspondence on CIHR's decision to ignore the misconduct. December, 2022.

[192] CIHR. "CIHR Grants and Awards Expenditures." Government of Canada. Accessed on February 11, 2023. https://cihr-irsc.gc.ca/e/51250.html.

[193] Justice Laws Website. "Canadian Institutes of Health Research Act." Government of Canada. Accessed February 12, 2023. https://laws-lois.justice.gc.ca/eng/acts/C-18.1/FullText.html.

[194] University of Toronto Libraries. "What counts as a scholarly source?" Utoronto.ca. Accessed on February 11, 2023. https://onesearch.library.utoronto.ca/faq/what-counts-scholarly-source.

[195] Collier, Roger. *CMAJ* (2015).

[196] Fisman et al., *MedRxiv* (2023 preprint).

[197] CIHR. "Project: Understanding, Forecasting and Communicating Risk During the COVID-19 Epidemic." Funding Decisions Database. Accessed on January 23, 2023. https://webapps.cihr-irsc.gc.ca/decisions/p/project_details.html?applId=422745&lang=en.

[198] Zamani, Farid. "Is Blackmail a Crime in Canada? | Penalty for Extortion." Zamani Law. October 21, 2019. https://zamani-law.com/extortion-a-primer/.

R v Alexander, 2005 CanLII 32566 (ON CA), [2005] OJ No 3777, per Doherty JA, at para 71 ("The section is aimed at those who would use coercion to overcome the free will of others for the purpose of extracting some gain:").

[199] R. v. McClure, 1957 CanLII 485 (MB CA), 22 WWR 167 (Man. C.A.), at p. 172. https://www.canlii.org/en/mb/mbca/doc/1957/1957canlii485/1957canlii485.html.

[200] Criminal Code Help. "Extortion or Blackmail Laws in Canada." Accessed on May 10, 2023. https://www.criminalcodehelp.ca/offences/against-property/extortion/.

[201] Brown, Catherine M., Johanna Vostok, Hillary Johnson et al. "Outbreak of SARS-CoV-2 Infections, Including COVID-19 Vaccine Breakthrough Infections, Associated with Large Public Gatherings — Barnstable County, Massachusetts, July 2021." *MMWR* (cdc.gov). August 6, 2021. 70(31);1059-1062. https://

www.cdc.gov/mmwr/volumes/70/wr/mm7031e2.htm.

[202] Subramanian, S.V., Kumar, A. "Increases in COVID-19 are unrelated to levels of vaccination across 68 countries and 2947 counties in the United States." *Eur J Epidemiol 36, 1237–1240.* September 30 2021. https://doi.org/10.1007/s10654-021-00808-7.

[203] Acharya, Charlotte B. et al. "Viral Load Among Vaccinated and Unvaccinated, Asymptomatic and Symptomatic Persons Infected With the SARS-CoV-2 Delta Variant." *Open Forum Infectious Diseases, Volume 9, Issue 5.* May 2022. https://doi.org/10.1093/ofid/ofac135.

[204] Bardosh K, de Figueiredo A, Gur-Arie R, et al. "The unintended consequences of COVID-19 vaccine policy: Why mandates, passports and restrictions may cause more harm than good." *BMJ Global Health.* May 26, 2022;7:e008684. https://doi.org/10.1136/bmjgh-2022-008684.

Singanayagam A, Hakki S, Dunning J, et al. "Community transmission and viral load kinetics of the SARS-CoV-2 delta (B.1.617.2) variant in vaccinated and unvaccinated individuals in the UK: a prospective, longitudinal, cohort study." *Lancet Infect Dis.* February 22, 2022:183–95. https://doi.org/10.1016/S1473-3099(21)00648-4.

[205] Kraaijeveld, S.R. "The Ethical Significance of Post-Vaccination COVID-19 Transmission Dynamics." *Bioethical Inquiry 20, 21–29.* March 2023. https://doi.org/10.1007/s11673-022-10223-6.

[206] Story, Alex. "France's Covid Passport Law Punishes Unvaccinated." *National Review.* January 24, 2022. https://www.nationalreview.com/2022/01/frances-vindictive-covid-strategy-make-life-miserable-for-the-unvaccinated/.

[207] Ellyatt, Holly. "Should we treat Covid like the flu? Europe is starting to think so." *CNBC.* January 12, 2022. https://www.cnbc.com/2022/01/12/should-we-treat-covid-like-the-flu-europe-is-starting-to-think-so.html.

[208] Aiello, Rachel. "Trudeau says Canadians 'angry' with anti-vaxxers." *CTV News.* January 5, 2022. https://www.ctvnews.ca/politics/canadians-are-angry-with-the-unvaccinated-trudeau-1.5728855.

[209] Hopper, Tristin. "FIRST READING: Canada's Omicron lockdowns among world's harshest." *National Post.* Jan 6, 2022. https://nationalpost.com/news/canada/first-reading-canadas-omicron-lockdowns-among-worlds-harshest.

[210] MacKinnon, Bobbi-Jean. "Province ponders proof of vaccination at liquor, cannabis stores." *CBC News.* January 14, 2022. https://www.cbc.ca/news/canada/new-brunswick/new-brunswick-covid-19-unvaccinated-restrictions-proof-liquor-cannabis-higgs-1.6314439.

[211] Stevenson, Verity and Isaac Olson. "Unvaccinated Quebecers will have to pay a health tax, Legault says." *CBC News.* January 11, 2022. https://www.cbc.ca/news/canada/montreal/unvaccinated-health-contribution-quebec-1.6311054.

[212] Blatchford, Andy. "Trudeau's own party is starting to turn on him over Covid restrictions." *Politico*. February 8, 2022. https://www.politico.com/news/2022/02/08/trudeau-lightbound-covid-restrictions-convoy-00006774.

[213] Treasury Board of Canada Secretariat. "Government of Canada to require vaccination of federal workforce and federally regulated transportation sector." Government of Canada. August 13, 2021. https://www.canada.ca/en/treasury-board-secretariat/news/2021/08/government-of-canada-to-require-vaccination-of-federal-workforce-and-federally-regulated-transportation-sector.html.

[214] Blatchford, Andy. "Trudeau injects vaccine hesitancy into spotlight of Canadian election." *Politico*. August 15, 2021. https://www.politico.com/news/2021/08/15/trudeau-canada-election-vaccine-hesitancy-504938.

[215] Global News. "[Video] Canada election: Trudeau slams protesters, says they're putting others at risk." August 31 2021. https://globalnews.ca/video/8156684/canada-election-trudeau-slams-protesters-says-theyre-putting-others-at-risk.

[216] Tasker, John Paul. "Trudeau promises $1B to help provinces pay for vaccine passports." *CBC News*. August 27, 2021. https://www.cbc.ca/news/politics/trudeau-promises-1b-vaccine-passports-1.6155618.

[217] Bingham, Jack. "Trudeau calls unvaccinated Canadians 'racists,' 'misogynists' in unhinged interview." *LifeSite News*. January 3, 2022. https://www.lifesitenews.com/news/trudeau-calls-unvaccinated-canadians-racists-misogynists-in-unhinged-interview/.

[218] Global News [Video]. "COVID-19: Trudeau says 'there will be consequences' for federal workers who are not fully vaccinated | Watch News Videos Online." August 17 2021. https://globalnews.ca/video/8119002/covid-19-trudeau-says-there-will-be-consequences-for-federal-workers-who-are-not-fully-vaccinated/.

Connolly, Amanda. "Trudeau doubles down on mandatory COVID-19 vaccines for domestic travel." *Global News*. August 18, 2021. https://globalnews.ca/news/8122807/canada-election-covid-19-madatory-vaccination/.

[219] Wherry, Aaron, Rosemary Barton, David Cochrane and Vassy Kapelos. "How the Liberals and New Democrats made a deal to preserve the minority government." *CBC News*. March 27, 2022. https://www.cbc.ca/news/politics/liberal-ndp-accord-confidence-supply-agreement-1.6397985.

[220] The Canadian Press. "Unvaccinated employees may not be eligible for EI: feds." Benefits Canada.com October 27, 2021. https://www.benefitscanada.com/human-resources/hr-law/unvaccinated-employees-may-not-be-eligible-for-ei-feds/.

[221] Palacios, Milagros and Ben Eisen. "Comparing Government and Private Sector Job Growth in the COVID-19 Era." Fraser Institute. August 2022. https://www.fraserinstitute.org/sites/default/files/comparing-government-and-private-

sector-job-growth-in-covid-19-era.pdf.

[222] Agility PR Solutions. "Top 10 Canadian Newspapers." Agilitypr.com. July 2022. https://www.agilitypr.com/resources/top-media-outlets/top-10-canadian-print-outlets/.

Yousif, Nadine. "When it comes to empathy for the unvaccinated, many of us aren't feeling it." *The Star*. August 26, 2021. https://www.thestar.com/news/gta/2021/08/26/when-it-comes-to-empathy-for-the-unvaccinated-many-of-us-arent-feeling-it.html.

[223] Bains, Camille. "'The ultimate selfishness': Doctors grow frustrated as anti-vaxxers protest hospitals." *Globalnews*. September 3, 2021. https://globalnews.ca/news/8164697/covid-coronavirus-doctors-frustrated-anti-vaccination/.

Arthur, Bruce. "The problem with anti-vaxxers is what to do about them." *The Toronto Star*. November 25, 2021. https://www.thestar.com/opinion/star-columnists/2021/11/25/the-problem-with-anti-vaxxers-is-what-to-do-about-them.html.

[224] CDC. "COVID-19 Pandemic Planning Scenarios." Accessed using the internet archive waybackmachine for May 31, 2020. http://web.archive.org/web/20200531215258/https://www.cdc.gov/coronavirus/2019-ncov/hcp/planning-scenarios.html.

[225] Ioannidis, John P A. "Infection fatality rate of COVID-19 inferred from seroprevalence data." CDC Bulletin. October 14, 2020. (Accessed using the waybackmachine). https://www.who.int/bulletin/online_first/BLT.20.265892.pdf.

[226] Canadian Human Rights Commission. "Vaccination policies and human rights: Frequently asked questions for employers and employees." October 21, 2021. https://www.chrc-ccdp.gc.ca/en/resources/vaccination-policies-and-human-rights-frequently-asked-questions-employers-and-employees.

[227] Government of Canada. "Canadian Human Rights Act." Accessed on June 11, 2023. https://laws-lois.justice.gc.ca/eng/acts/h-6/FullText.html.

[228] BC's Office of the Human Rights Commissioner. "A human rights approach to proof of vaccination during the COVID-19 pandemic." Accessed on June 11, 2023. https://bchumanrights.ca/publications/vaccination/.

[229] Alberta Human Rights Commission. "COVID-19 vaccine mandates and proof of vaccination." Revised December 15, 2022. Accessed on June 20, 2023. https://albertahumanrights.ab.ca/covid/Pages/vaccines.aspx.

[230] Newfoundland and Labrador Human Rights Commission. "COVID-19 and Human Rights - Best Practices." thinkhumanrights.ca Accessed on April 30, 2023. https://thinkhumanrights.ca/human-rights-and-covid-19-best-practices/.

[231] BC Center for Disease Control. "Vaccine Considerations." Accessed on April 30, 2023. http://www.bccdc.ca/health-info/diseases-conditions/covid-19/covid-19-vaccine/vaccine-considerations.

[232] French, Janet. "New Alberta premier says unvaccinated 'most discriminated against group' after swearing-in." *CBC News.* Oct 11, 2022. https://www.cbc.ca/news/canada/edmonton/new-alberta-premier-says-unvaccinated-most-discriminated-against-group-after-swearing-in-1.6612767.

[233] Ontario Human Rights Commission. "COVID-19 and Ontario's Human Rights Code – Questions and Answers." Accessed on June 24, 2022. https://www.ohrc.on.ca/en/news_centre/covid-19-and-ontario%E2%80%99s-human-rights-code-%E2%80%93-questions-and-answers.

[234] Wyton, Moira. "Regulated health professionals no longer required to disclose COVID-19 vaccination status in B.C." *CBC News.* Jul 18, 2023. https://www.cbc.ca/news/canada/british-columbia/bc-order-health-professionals-covid19-vaccine-reporting-1.6909223.

CharityVillage. "Job Notice: Policy and Research Specialist - Posted July 13, 2023." Accessed on July 29, 2023. https://charityvillage.com/jobs/policy-and-research-specialist-in-ottawa-ontario-ca/.

Municipality of Middlesex Centre. "Job Notice: Community Services - Facility Attendant Ilderton & Komoka Arenas - Career Portal, posted July 24, 2023." Dayforcehcm.com. Accessed on July 29, 2023. https://can231.dayforcehcm.com/CandidatePortal/en-US/middlesex/Posting/View/276.

Simplyhired.ca. "Care Coordinator - Home and Community Care Support Services Central East | Scarborough, ON – Posted July 27, 2023." Accessed on July 29, 2023. https://www.simplyhired.ca/job/lrF3u1j8ynnZbGzQyXQyALwBdgwP2HPH2o_l2--ojXJ1lwB9i6zRKA.

RNCareers. "Registered Nurse - Emergency job with Orilla Soldiers' Memorial Hospital | 2064552." Accessed on July 29, 2023. https://www.rncareers.ca/job/2064552/registered-nurse-emergency.

[235] Doshi (BMJ, 2020); Pfizer (FDA Briefing, 2020); Government of Canada (Regulatory Decisions, 2021).

[236] Palmer Michael, Sucharit Bhakdi and Stefan Hockertz. "Expert evidence regarding Comirnaty (Pfizer) COVID-19 mRNA Vaccine for children." Doctors for COVID Ethics. (doctors4covidethics.org). July 3, 2021. https://doctors4covidethics.org/expert-evidence-regarding-comirnaty-covid-19-mrna-vaccine-for-children/.

[237] Palmer, Bhakdi and Hockertz (EU Testimony, July 2021).

[238] Health Canada. "Health Canada authorizes first COVID-19 vaccine." December 9, 2020. https://www.canada.ca/en/health-canada/news/2020/12/health-canada-authorizes-first-covid-19-vaccine0.html.

[239] Petkov, Hristo. "The challenges of the global distribution of COVID-19 vaccines." Maersk. January 29 2021. https://www.maersk.com/news/articles/2021/01/29/the-challenges-of-the-covid-19-vaccine-global-distribution.

Palmer, Michael and Jonathan Gilthorpe. "COVID-19 mRNA vaccines contain excessive quantities of bacterial DNA: evidence and implications." Doctors for COVID Ethics. April 5, 2023. https://doctors4covidethics.org/covid-19-mrna-vaccines-contain-excessive-quantities-of-bacterial-dna-evidence-and-implications/.

Bruce Yu Y, Taraban MB, Briggs KT. "All vials are not the same: Potential role of vaccine quality in vaccine adverse reactions." *Vaccine*. 2021 Oct 29;39(45): 6565-6569. https://doi.org/10.1016/j.vaccine.2021.09.065. Epub 2021 Oct 6. PMID: 34625289; PMCID: PMC8492451.

Mendez, Rich. "Japan halts 1.6 million Moderna Covid vaccine doses over contamination concerns." *CNBC*. August 26 2021. https://www.cnbc.com/2021/08/26/japan-pulls-1point6-million-moderna-vaccine-doses-over-contamination-concerns-.html.

Banco, Erin and Sarah Owermohle. "Emergent's Covid vaccine problems more extensive than previously known." *Politico*. May 10, 2022. https://www.politico.com/news/2022/05/10/emergent-covid-vaccine-problems-00031266.

Stolberg, Sheryl Gay; Chris Hamby; and Sharon LaFraniere. "Emergent Hid Evidence of Covid Vaccine Problems at Plant, Report Says." *The New York Times*. May 10, 2022. https://www.nytimes.com/2022/05/10/us/politics/emergent-fda-vaccine-covid-contaminated.html.

Blackwell, Tom. "More than half Canada's AstraZeneca vaccine came from U.S. plant accused of quality-control problems." *National Post*. April 23, 2021. https://nationalpost.com/news/canada/more-than-half-canadas-astrazeneca-vaccine-came-from-u-s-plant-accused-by-fda-of-quality-control-problems.

Neustaeter, Brooklyn. "Health Canada holding J&J COVID-19 vaccines over possible quality control issue." *CTV News*. April 30, 2021. https://www.ctvnews.ca/health/coronavirus/health-canada-holding-j-j-covid-19-vaccines-over-possible-quality-control-issue-1.5409817.

National Citizens Inquiry. "Dr. Laura Braden, Day 3 Truro Hearing, National Citizens Inquiry." NCI (rumble.com). March 27, 2023. https://rumble.com/v2f2d4g-truro-hearing-day-1-expert-witness-dr-laura-braden.html.

[240] National Citizens Inquiry. "Shawn Buckley - The Political Approval of the Covid Vaccine: A Constitutional Lawyer's Perspective | Quebec City Day Two." NCI (rumble.com). May 12, 2023. https://rumble.com/v2nowc2-shawn-buckley-shares-his-legal-perspective-on-health-canada-measures-quebec.html.

[241] Health Canada. "Regulatory Decision Summary - COMIRNATY." September 16, 2021. https://covid-vaccine.canada.ca/info/regulatory-decision-summary-detail.html?linkID=RDS00856.

Government of Canada. "Drug and vaccine authorizations for COVID-19: Authorized drugs, vaccines and expanded indications." Canada.ca. Accessed on

June 8, 2023. https://www.canada.ca/en/health-canada/services/drugs-health-products/covid19-industry/drugs-vaccines-treatments/authorization/list-drugs.html.

[242] House of Commons of Canada. "Evidence - PACP (44-1) - No. 50." February 13, 2023. https://www.ourcommons.ca/DocumentViewer/en/44-1/PACP/meeting-50/evidence.

[243] Government of Canada. "Stop illegal marketing of drugs and devices." Accessed on June 14, 2023. https://www.canada.ca/en/health-canada/services/drugs-health-products/marketing-drugs-devices/illegal-marketing/stop.html.

[244] Government of Canada. "Beware of these illegal marketing practices - Canada.ca." Accessed on June 14, 2023. https://www.canada.ca/en/health-canada/services/drugs-health-products/marketing-drugs-devices/illegal-marketing/practices.html.

[245] Doshi, Peter. "Covid-19 vaccines: In the rush for regulatory approval, do we need more data?" *BMJ*. May 18 2021;373:n1244. https://doi.org/10.1136/bmj.n1244.

Lenzer, Jeanne. "Covid-19: Should vaccine trials be unblinded?" *BMJ*. December 29 2020; 371. https://doi.org/10.1136/bmj.m4956.

[246] MacDonald, Noni, Shelly A. McNeil, Jeannette Comeau, Shawn Harmon, Eve Dubé and Lucie M. Bucci. "Surveillance for COVID-19 Vaccine Effectiveness and Serious Adverse Events Following Immunization." CANVax. September 21, 2020. https://canvax.ca/brief/surveillance-covid-19-vaccine-effectiveness-and-serious-adverse-events-following-immunization.

[247] Comité sur l'immunisation du Québec. "Administration of COVID-19 booster doses: Recommendations for winter and spring 2023." INSPQ. December 21, 2022. https://www.inspq.qc.ca/sites/default/files/publications/3284-covid-19-booster-doses-winter-spring-2023.pdf.

Statistics Canada (2021). "Provisional death counts and excess mortality, January 2020 to February 2021 [Internet]." The Daily. May 14, 2021 [Accessed on June 27, 2023]. Available from: https://www150.statcan.gc.ca/n1/daily-quotidien/210514/dq210514c-eng.htm.

[248] CDC. "COVID-19 Provisional Counts - Weekly Updates by Select Demographic and Geographic Characteristics." Accessed on June 28, 2023. https://www.cdc.gov/nchs/nvss/vsrr/covid_weekly/index.htm#Comorbidities.

[249] Public Health Agency of Canada. "News Release: Government of Canada supports projects to encourage vaccine uptake in Canada." February 2, 2021. https://www.canada.ca/en/public-health/news/2021/02/government-of-canada-supports-projects-to-encourage-vaccine-uptake-in-canada.html.

Dzsurdzsa, Cosmin. "Feds have spent $139 million to date on Covid ad campaigns." *True North News*. February 6, 2023. https://tnc.news/2023/02/06/covid-ad-campaigns/.

Government of Canada. "Annual report on Government of Canada Advertising Activities 2021 to 2022." Accessed on June 28, 2023. https://www.tpsgc-pwgsc.gc.ca/pub-adv/rapports-reports/documents/rapport-annuel-annual-report-2021-2022-eng.pdf.

Government of Canada. "Annual report on Government of Canada Advertising Activities 2020 to 2021." Accessed on June 28, 2023. https://www.tpsgc-pwgsc.gc.ca/pub-adv/rapports-reports/documents/rapport-annuel-annual-report-2020-2021-eng.pdf.

Public Health Agency of Canada. "Government of Canada launches new "Ripple Effect" advertising campaign to encourage COVID-19 vaccination." Government of Canada. May 17, 2021. https://www.canada.ca/en/public-health/news/2021/05/government-of-canada-launches-new-ripple-effect-advertising-campaign-to-encourage-covid-19-vaccination.html.

Franklin, Michael. "Changing messaging the real challenge for Alberta's vaccine ad campaign, expert says." *CTV News*. May 13, 2021. https://calgary.ctvnews.ca/your-vaccine-is-your-ticket-alberta-government-pushes-vaccination-through-ad-campaign-1.5426962.

[250] Tadrous, Mina , "Assessing the Sensitivity of the Canadian Adverse Event Following Immunization Surveillance System (CAEFISS)" (2010). Theses and Dissertations (ETD). Paper 262. http://dx.doi.org/ 10.21007/etd.cghs.2010.0309.

Blumenthal, K.G. et al. "Acute Allergic Reactions to mRNA COVID-19 Vaccines." *JAMA*. April 20, 2021;325(15):1562-1565. https://doi.org/10.1001/jama.2021.3976.

[251] Aziz, Saba. "With millions of COVID-19 vaccine doses wasted, has Canada kept its donation promises? – National." *Global News*. December 9, 2022. https://globalnews.ca/news/9337650/canada-covid-vaccine-wastage-donations/.

Osman, Laura. "Expired COVID-19 vaccines to cost Canada $1 billion: AG report." *National Post*. Dec 06, 2022. https://nationalpost.com/news/most-unused-covid-19-vaccines-will-expire-at-the-end-of-the-year-auditor-general.

[252] Government of Canada. "Canada's aid and development assistance in response to COVID 19." International.gc.ca. Accessed on June 28, 2023. https://www.international.gc.ca/world-monde/issues_development-enjeux_developpement/global_health-sante_mondiale/response_covid-19_reponse.aspx?lang=eng.

[253] Pfizer-BioNTech. "COVID-19 mRNA vaccine(nucleoside modified)Periodic Safety Update Report (PSUR) 3." August 18, 2022. https://tkp.at/wp-content/uploads/2023/03/3.PSUR-1.pdf.

Horowitz, Daniel. "Confidential Pfizer document shows the company observed 1.6 million adverse events covering nearly every organ system." *Conservative Review*. June 14, 2023. https://www.conservativereview.com/horowitz-confidential-pfizer-document-shows-the-company-observed-1-6-million-adverse-events-covering-nearly-every-organ-system-2661316948.html.

[254] The College of Physicians and Surgeons Manitoba. "CPSM Vaccines FAQs.pdf." CPSM. September 30, 2021. https://cpsm.mb.ca/assets/COVID19/CPSM%20Vaccines%20FAQs.pdf.

The College of Physicians and Surgeons of Ontario. "COVID-19 Exemption Requests – eDialogue." CPSO. September 22, 2021. https://dialogue.cpso.on.ca/2021/09/covid-19-exemption-requests/.

[255] Ahmed, Alex Anas. "1996 report says Canada's Health Department found 'immunization was not mandatory.'" *The Post Millennial*. Oct 16, 2021. https://thepostmillennial.com/canadas-health-department-mandatory-immunization.

[256] Ahmed, Alex Anas. "1996 report says Canada's Health Department found 'immunization was not mandatory.'" *The Post Millennial*. Oct 16, 2021. https://thepostmillennial.com/canadas-health-department-mandatory-immunization.

[257] Radwanski, George. "Speech: Opening Statement regarding Bill C-217 (Blood Samples Act) - February 21, 2002." Office of the Privacy Commissioner of Canada. February 21, 2002. https://www.priv.gc.ca/en/opc-actions-and-decisions/advice-to-parliament/archive/02_05_a_020222/.

[258] Nielsen, Kevin. "Ontario courts shutting down in a bid to slow coronavirus." *Global News*. March 16, 2020. https://globalnews.ca/news/6683865/ontario-courts-coronavirus.

Raymer, Elizabeth. "Courts across Canada restrict access or suspend operations due to COVID-19." *Canadian Lawyer*. March 16 2020. https://www.canadianlawyermag.com/news/general/courts-across-canada-restrict-access-or-suspend-operations-due-to-covid-19/327534.

[259] Government of Canada. "Chief Justice of Canada and Minister of Justice Launch Action Committee on Court Operations in Response to COVID-19." May 8, 2020. https://www.canada.ca/en/department-justice/news/2020/05/chief-justice-of-canada-and-minister-of-justice-launch-action-committee-on-court-operations-in-response-to-covid-19.html.

[260] Office of the Commissioner for Federal Judicial Affairs Canada. "Action Committee on Court Operations in Response to COVID-19." Government of Canada. Accessed on June 14, 2023. https://fja.gc.ca/COVID-19/reference-eng.html.

[261] Schmitz, Cristin. "Federal Court becomes first known court to disclose COVID-19 vaccination status of its judges." *Law360 Canada*. September 3, 2021. https://www.law360.ca/articles/29570/federal-court-becomes-first-known-court-to-disclose-covid-19-vaccination-status-of-its-judges.

[262] Federal Court of Canada. Twitter (@FedCourt_CAN_en). September 2, 2021.

[263] Schmitz, Cristin. "Supreme Court mandates COVID jabs for in-court staff;

Federal C.A. won't disclose COVID policies." *Law360 Canada*. September 07, 2021. https://www.law360.ca/articles/29605/supreme-court-mandates-covid-jabs-for-in-court-staff-federal-c-a-won-t-disclose-covid-policies.

[264] Harper v. Canada (Attorney General), 2000 SCC 57, [2000] 2 S.C.R. 764. CanLII. November 10, 2000. https://www.canlii.org/en/ca/scc/doc/2000/2000scc57/2000scc57.html.

[265] RJR--MacDonald Inc. v. Canada (Attorney General), 1994 CanLII 117 (SCC), [1994] 1 S.C.R. 311, at pp. 348-49.

[266] R. v. J.M., 2021 ONCA 150. CanLII. https://canlii.ca/t/jdnw3. Retrieved on 2023-06-16.

[267] M.M. v. W.A.K., 2022 ONSC 4580. CanLII. https://canlii.ca/t/jr8xb. Retrieved on 2023-06-15.

Alexander, Russell. "Court Refuses to Take Judicial Notice of COVID-19 Vaccine 'Facts.'" CanLII Connects. August 22, 2022. https://canliiconnects.org/en/commentaries/89421.

[268] Canada (Attorney General) v. Bedford. [2013] 3 SCR 1101 at paragraph 127. https://scc-csc.lexum.com/scc-csc/scc-csc/en/item/13389/index.do.

[269] Government of Canada. "Charterpedia - Section 7 – Life, liberty and security of the person." Justice.gc.ca. Accessed on April 9, 2023. https://justice.gc.ca/eng/csj-sjc/rfc-dlc/ccrf-ccdl/check/art7.html.

[270] Government of Canada. "Policy on COVID-19 Vaccination for the Core Public Administration Including the Royal Canadian Mounted Police." Accessed on August 6, 2023. https://www.tbs-sct.canada.ca/pol/doc-eng.aspx?id=32694&section=html.

[271] Prime Minister of Canada. "Prime Minister announces mandatory vaccination for the federal workforce and federally regulated transportation sectors." pm.gc.ca. October 6, 2021. https://www.pm.gc.ca/en/news/news-releases/2021/10/06/prime-minister-announces-mandatory-vaccination-federal-workforce-and.

[272] Ioannidis, 2020.

[273] Statistics Canada, 2021.

[274] Schwab, Constantin, Lisa Maria Domke, Laura Hartmann, Albrecht Stenzinger, Thomas Longerich and Peter Schirmacher. "Autopsy-based histopathological characterization of myocarditis after anti-SARS-CoV-2-vaccination." Clin Res Cardiol. 2023 Mar;112(3):431-440. https://doi.org/10.1007/s00392-022-02129-5. Epub November 27, 2022.

Margulis, Jennifer and Joe Wang. "People Died From mRNA-Vaccine-Damaged Hearts, New Peer-Reviewed German Study Provides Direct Evidence." *Epoch Times*. December 12, 2022. https://www.theepochtimes.com/health/people-died-from-mrna-vaccine-damaged-hearts-new-peer-reviewed-german-study-provides-direct-evidence_4919662.html.

Chevassut, Tim, Beverley J. Hunt and Sue Pavord. "VITT, COVID-19 and the Expert Haematology Panel: The story of how the UK responded to emerging cases of vaccine-induced immune thrombocytopenia and thrombosis during the vaccination programme | RCP Journals." *Clinical Medicine Journal.* November 2021. DOI: https://doi.org/10.7861/clinmed.2021-0488.

[275] UKHSA. "COVID-19 vaccine surveillance report Week 42, UK Health Security Agency." OCT 21, 2021. https://assets.publishing.service.gov.uk/government/uploads/system/uploads/attachment_data/file/1027511/Vaccine-surveillance-report-week-42.pdf.

[276] R. v. Malmo-Levine; R. v. Caine [2003] 3 S.C.R. 571 at paragraph 98. https://scc-csc.lexum.com/scc-csc/scc-csc/en/item/2109/index.do.

[277] Canada (Attorney General) v. Bedford. [2013] 3 SCR 1101 at paragraphs 125-126. https://scc-csc.lexum.com/scc-csc/scc-csc/en/item/13389/index.do.

[278] Lowe, Julie and Samuel E Trosow. "Surfing the Fourth Wave: Riding out a Charter Challenge to University and College Vaccination Mandates." Canadian Legal Information Institute, 2021 CanLIIDocs 1946. https://canlii.ca/t/tb1c. Retrieved on 2023-04-02.

Hogg, Peter W. "Constitutional Law of Canada, (2019 Student Edition, Thomson Reuters) at 38-49." (as cited by Lowe and Trosow).

[279] Charkaoui v. Canada (Citizenship and Immigration), [2007] 1 S.C.R. 350, at paragraphs 66. https://scc-csc.lexum.com/scc-csc/scc-csc/en/item/2345/index.do.

[280] National Post. "Trudeau's COVID-19 vaccine comments draw angry response from foes." April 26, 2023. https://nationalpost.com/news/canada/trudeau-says-he-didnt-force-anyone-to-get-vaccinated-all-the-incentives-were-there-to-encourage-canadians.

[281] Singh v. Minister of Employment and Immigration, [1985] 1 S.C.R. 177 at para 103. https://scc-csc.lexum.com/scc-csc/scc-csc/en/item/39/index.do.

[282] Government of Canada. "Government of Canada to require vaccination of federal workforce and federally regulated transportation sector." Accessed September 21, 2022. https://www.canada.ca/en/treasury-board-secretariat/news/2021/08/government-of-canada-to-require-vaccination-of-federal-workforce-and-federally-regulated-transportation-sector.html.

[283] Palacios, Milagros and Ben Eisen. *Fraser Institute* (August 2022).

[284] Hopper, Tristin. "FIRST READING: The evidence against Trudeau's claim he didn't 'force' vaccination." *SaltWire.* May 1, 2023. https://www.saltwire.com/atlantic-canada/opinion/first-reading-the-evidence-against-trudeaus-claim-he-didnt-force-vaccination-100848956/.

[285] CMPA. "Consent: A guide for Canadian physicians." Accessed on August 7, 2023. https://www.cmpa-acpm.ca/en/advice-publications/handbooks/consent-a-

guide-for-canadian-physicians#.

[286] The Canadian Press. "Unvaccinated employees may not be eligible for EI: feds." Benefits Canada.com. October 27, 2021 https://www.benefitscanada.com/human-resources/hr-law/unvaccinated-employees-may-not-be-eligible-for-ei-feds.

[287] Irwin Toy Ltd. v. Quebec (Attorney General) [1989] 1 SCR 927 at 1003. Accessed on August 7, 2023. https://scc-csc.lexum.com/scc-csc/scc-csc/en/item/443/index.do.

Gosselin v. Québec (Attorney General) 2002 SCC 84 at paragraph 80. Accessed on August 7, 2023. https://scc-csc.lexum.com/scc-csc/scc-csc/en/item/2027/index.do.

As cited by Government of Canada. https://justice.gc.ca/eng/csj-sjc/rfc-dlc/ccrf-ccdl/check/art7.html.

[288] KCY AT LAW. "Workplace Replacements & Disciplinary Suspensions in Canada." Accessed on June 19, 2023. https://www.kcyatlaw.ca/workplace-suspensions-in-canada/.

[289] Verlint, Monty and Rhonda B. Levy. "Court confirms unions must challenge vaccination policies before labour arbitrators." HRD Canada (hcamag.com) December 3, 2021. https://www.hcamag.com/ca/specialization/employment-law/court-confirms-unions-must-challenge-vaccination-policies-before-labour-arbitrators/318787.

Vaughan, Eleanor A. and Rachel M. Counsell. "Court Denies Injunction Motions and Allows Mandatory Vaccination Policies to be Implemented." Hicksmorley.com. November 20, 2021. https://hicksmorley.com/2021/11/20/court-denies-injunction-motions-and-allows-mandatory-vaccination-policies-to-be-implemented/.

[290] Bundale, Brett. "Challenges to workplace vaccine mandates being tossed out, legal experts say." *CBC News*. February 7, 2022. https://www.cbc.ca/news/business/vaccine-mandates-1.6342193.

[291] Toronto Professional Fire Fighters' Association, I.A.A.F. Local 3888 and City of Toronto (Re: Mandatory Vaccine Policy Grievance, Para 232). Arbitrator: Derek L. Rogers. August 26, 2022. https://hicksmorley.com/wp-content/uploads/2022/09/TPFFA-and-City-of-Toronto-Rogers-26-August-2022.pdf.

[292] City of Toronto and Toronto Civic Employees' Union, CUPE, Local 416 (In the matter of a policy grievance concerning a mandatory vaccine policy, para 47). Arbitrator Robert J. Herman. November 21, 2022.

[293] Syndicat des métallos, section locale 2008 c. Procureur général du Canada, 2022 QCCS 2455 (para 49, 175). https://www.canlii.org/fr/qc/qccs/doc/2022/2022qccs2455/2022qccs2455.html.

[294] FCA Canada Inc. v Unifor, Locals 195, 444, 1285, 2022 CanLII 52913 (ON LA).

CanLII. https://canlii.ca/t/jpvl4. Retrieved on 2023-06-19.

[295] Horwood, Matthew. "EXCLUSIVE: Canadian Military's COVID Vaccine Mandate Violated Charter Rights, Grievance Review Committee Finds." *Epoch Times*. June 15, 2023. https://www.theepochtimes.com/exclusive-militarys-covid-vaccine-mandate-violated-charter-rights-grievance-review-committee-finds_5332851.html.

[296] Ritchie, Sarah. "External review found military's COVID-19 vaccine policy violated Charter of Rights." *CBC News*. August 1, 2023. https://www.cbc.ca/news/politics/military-covid-19-vaccine-policy-charter-1.6924862.

[297] Wilson, Keith, Allison Pejovic and Eva Chipiuk. "2022-08-10 Federal Travel Mandate Factum (FINAL)." Wilson Law Office & JCCF. August 9, 2022. https://www.jccf.ca/wp-content/uploads/2022/08/2022-08-10-Federal-Travel-Mandate-Factum-FINAL_Redacted.pdf.

[298] Subramanya, Rupa. "Court Documents Reveal Canada's Travel Ban Had No Scientific Basis." *Global Research*. August 4, 2022. https://www.globalresearch.ca/court-documents-reveal-canada-travel-ban-had-no-scientific-basis/5788833.

[299] Joy, Lisa. "Brian Peckford and Maxime Bernier may appeal the decision." *SaskToday.ca*. October 24, 2022. https://www.sasktoday.ca/north/local-news/federal-court-tosses-constitutional-challenge-to-travel-ban-5998811.

[300] Justice Centre for Constitutional Freedoms. "Bernier, Peckford file written appeal argument on "mootness" at Federal Court of Appeal." JCCF.ca. April 24, 2023. https://www.jccf.ca/bernier-peckford-file-written-appeal-argument-on-mootness-at-federal-court-of-appeal/.

[301] CPAC. "[Video] Justin Trudeau holds rally in Sudbury." August 31, 2021. (10:04 minute mark)." YouTube. https://www.youtube.com/watch?v=v6Sx8Mw0CmA.

[302] United Nations Population Fund. "Bodily autonomy: Busting 7 myths that undermine individual rights and freedoms." UNFPA. April 14, 2021. https://www.unfpa.org/news/bodily-autonomy-busting-7-myths-undermine-individual-rights-and-freedoms.

[303] Zimonjic, Peter. "Provinces could make vaccination mandatory, says federal health minister." *CBC News*. January 7, 2022. https://www.cbc.ca/news/politics/duclos-mandatory-vaccination-policies-on-way-1.6307398.

[304] Lowrie, Morgan (Canadian Press, 2022).

[305] Hart, Robert (Forbes, 2022).

[306] Macintyre, Ben. *Operation Mincemeat: How a Dead Man and a Bizarre Plan Fooled the Nazis and Assured an Allied Victory.* Bloomsbury. May 4, 2010.

[307] CDC. "COVID-19 Pandemic Planning Scenarios." Accessed using the internet archive waybackmachine for May 31, 2020. http://web.archive.org/web/20200531215258/https://www.cdc.gov/coronavirus/2019-ncov/hcp/planning-scenarios.html.

[308] Ioannidis, John P A. "Infection fatality rate of COVID-19 inferred from seroprevalence data." CDC Bulletin. October 14, 2020. (Accessed using the waybackmachine). https://www.who.int/bulletin/online_first/BLT.20.265892.pdf.

[309] Croft, Ashley. "Report for the Scottish COVID-19 Inquiry." Scottish COVID-19 Inquiry. July 10, 2023. https://www.covid19inquiry.scot/hearings/epidemiology-presentation.

Dockrell DH, Sundar S, Angus BJ. Infectious disease. In: Penman ID, Ralston SH, Strachan MW, Hobson RP, eds. Davidson's principles and practice of medicine. 24th ed. London: Elsevier, 2022.

[310] Global News. "[Video] Coronavirus: Trudeau tells UN conference that pandemic provided 'opportunity for a reset.'" September 2020. https://www.youtube.com/watch?v=n2fp0Jeyjvw.

Lao, David. "COVID-19 opened 'window of political opportunity' to implement national childcare: Freeland – National." *Global News*. April 8, 2021. https://globalnews.ca/news/7747194/chrystia-freeland-budget-canada-childcare/.

Murphy, Rex. "Chrystia Freeland's 'epiphany' that COVID-19 is an 'opportunity' — that's pretty dark." *National Post*. April 15, 2021. https://nationalpost.com/opinion/rex-murphy-chrystia-freelands-epiphany-that-covid-19-is-an-opportunity-is-actually-pretty-dark.

ABOUT THE AUTHOR

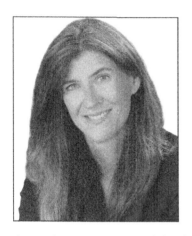

Regina holds a PhD in Statistics from the University of Western Ontario with a strong background in the sciences. She has served as a consultant to medical practitioners, social scientists and various levels of government. She also served as the principal statistician for an Ottawa-based economics consulting firm that specialized in econometrics, program evaluation, business case development and risk-benefit-options analysis.

As project manager and lead analyst, Dr. Watteel routinely engaged with stakeholder groups to deliver comprehensive solutions from early needs assessments and metrics development through to data collection, performance measurement, statistical analysis and the dissemination of findings, including implications and limitations. She has taught both undergraduate and graduate level university courses in multivariate statistical analysis, data analysis and engineering statistics.

Dr. Watteel's career path took a dramatic turn following a motor vehicle accident in which a substance impaired driver plowed into her while she was putting groceries in the trunk of her vehicle. Ultimately, Dr. Watteel stepped down from her position to focus on rehabilitation, health and her three children. She also took the opportunity to branch out and pursue aspirations in the publishing business. During the pandemic, concerns over the censorship of important scientific information and a government course of action that seemed to be moving in a direction of maximal harm and risk prompted a passionate return as a statistical sleuth.

Since March 2020, Regina N. Watteel has monitored the evolving world-wide pandemic data, government responses and emerging scientific findings. Early on, it became apparent to Dr. Watteel that the government's actions were not based on sound decision-making practices and were at odds with their own risk management framework, which they appeared to have abandoned completely. She has been outspoken about the need for transparency and the importance of adhering to a rational, evidence-based approach that is open to scrutiny.

Printed in Great Britain
by Amazon

56138288R00136